**Semyon Krewer is the author of THE ARTHRITIS EXERCISE BOOK**

# Help for Your ARTHRITIC HAND

New exercises, hints, and aids for daily living to help prevent needless disability

Semyon Krewer

In collaboration with Ann Edgar, R.P.T.

Foreword by Samuel S. Sverdlik, M.D.
Director, Dept. of Rehabilitation Medicine
St. Vincent's Hospital and Medical Center of New York

Cornerstone Library
Published by Simon & Schuster NEW YORK

Dedicated to my wife, Elsa,
who helped to construct the Hand Gym

Sections of this book were previously published as part of *The Arthritis Exercise Book*


Published by Cornerstone Library
A Simon & Schuster Division of Gulf & Western Corporation
Simon & Schuster Building
1230 Avenue of the Americas
New York, New York 10020

CORNERSTONE LIBRARY and colophon are trademarks of Simon & Schuster, registered in the U.S. Patent and Trademark Office

Manufactured in the United States of America

10 9 8 7 6 5 4 3 2 1

ISBN 0-346-12565-0

# Contents

# A NOTE TO THE READER

The exercises in this book are designed to maintain and increase your strength, flexibility, and endurance. The exercises can be considered *preventive,* since they may help to delay the onset of symptoms of osteoarthritis. If rheumatoid arthritis has occurred, the exercises can be considered *therapeutic*.

If you are under the care of a physician for the treatment of arthritis, please consult him or her about the exercises that seem best for you.

**IMPORTANT WARNING:** The exercises in this book are not meant to be carried out by persons with severe crippling from rheumatoid arthritis. It would be painful and even harmful for such persons to attempt to use the Hand Gym.

All exercises in this book are designed to incur practically no pain that would linger for any length of time. If pain should follow from any particular exercise, that exercise may not be appropriate for you; consult your physician about it. Your doctor can prescribe a personalized program for you, which may contain some of the exercises in this book.

If you have rheumatoid arthritis, please do not consider exercises and physical therapy as exclusive treatment for your condition. These are very important modalities which are only part of an overall medical treatment program consisting of medication, a balanced mix of rest and activity, and physical therapy.

S. K.

# Medical Foreword

Reading this book with a doctor's bias made me aware of the truth to the dictum that every good physician listens to his patient. Patients with chronic diseases and disabilities who are continuously faced with coping with problems will always come up with solutions or adaptations that only someone living with the problem could evolve.

Every patient also brings his or her background to these challenges. An intelligent individual will bring together his education, faith, energy and dedication in dealing with problems. Semyon Krewer is such a man.

He brings his engineering background, curiosity, scholarship and, above all, the maturity to seek help from others. He applies common sense in making a judgment and acting upon recommendations. He doesn't see disaster in having rheumatoid arthritis, nor does he see confusion, ignorance or conflict in legitimate differences of treatment.

The uncertainty of response to medication and treatment of arthritis is further complicated by the difficulty in getting people to appreciate the need for rest, exercise and physical/occupational therapy. The patient's role is critical to the success of this effort. More particularly is this true when treating the arthritic hand, and most telling with the patient with rheumatoid arthritis. This book, which reflects the personal experience of a man who is living with the problem and has come to grips with it, is most striking by the informative manner in which it deals with this special problem.

The progression of hand disablement is one of the most frustrating and painful encounters a patient, his family and physician can experience. To control the disability, prevent or slow its evolution, is an achievement to be praised highly. The Hand Gym is a practical device that can be of great value in alleviating or limiting hand disability.

I recommend this volume to patients, their families and health professionals who are interested in reading about how a patient can deal with a very difficult problem and come to terms with it. It is a practical and realistic statement which anyone encountering hand disablement will find helpful and hopeful.

*Samuel S. Sverdlik, M.D.*
*Director, Department of Rehabilitation Medicine*
*St. Vincent's Hospital and Medical Center of New York*

# Acknowledgments

Some years ago I became involved in the Student Help for the Elderly program at Columbia University—first as one of those benefiting from the help it provided, and later as a member of the Board of Student Help. It seemed to me that the program could be more effective if the students were better informed about suitable exercises for the elderly, especially those with arthritis. My suggestion to this effect was well received, but we could not at that time find any literature that furnished detailed instructions.

The local chapter of the Arthritis Foundation referred us to Ann Edgar, chief physical therapist at the arthritis clinic at Columbia Presbyterian Hospital, New York, who instructed some of the students in home exercise assistance. I saw then the need for a book containing detailed, well-illustrated exercises and instructions—especially for isometric exercises, which are frequently recommended but almost nowhere properly described. This book will, I hope, answer that need.

I owe a debt of gratitude also to Dr. Edward Lowman, Clinical Director of the Institute of Rehabilitation Medicine (I.R.M.), New York University Medical Center, for sponsoring a clinical evaluation of the device called the Hand Gym, which I designed for my own use. One outcome of the study was a set of detailed instructions for using the Hand Gym, prepared by Doris Bens, O.T.R., of the occupational therapy department of the Institute, under the direction of Sophie Chiotelis, O.T.R. Dr. Lowman facilitated my carrying out myographic research (measurement of electrical impulses accompanying muscle contractions), which enabled me to design isometric exercises for the Hand Gym. Muriel Zimmerman, O.T.R., at I.R.M. introduced me to the excellent collection of self-help aids which she assembled.

I wish to thank Dr. Samuel Sverdlik, chairman of the rehabilitation medicine department at St. Vincent's Hospital, New York City, for supervising a clinical study of twenty-three arthritic patients using the Hand Gym that included a four-year follow-up. This work convinced me that a well-illustrated exercise system could effectively be carried out at home.

I am grateful to Dr. Valery Lanyi of the arthritis clinic at Bellevue Hospital, New York City, for encouraging me to pursue my analysis of the interconnection between lymphatic function, arthritic symptoms, and modalities of physical therapy.

In designing the exercises, I had in mind also the words of caution I have heard from many rheumatologists, notably Dr. George Ehrlich of the Hahnemann Medical College in Philadelphia, about the current popularity of jogging and tennis. Persons prone to osteoarthritis may hasten the onset of this condition by engaging in sports of this sort, which place severe stress on the weight-bearing joints.

For help in analyzing certain aspects of physiology and anatomy, I am grateful to my daughter Julie Ann Krewer.

I thank my friend Charles C. Bennett for helping me to present new ideas in physical therapy for arthritics to the profession and, once these approaches were found to be beneficial, for helping me to make this information more widely available to the public.

Finally, I wish to acknowledge the careful work of Lynn Thompson Welch in preparing the numerous illustrations for this book which promote hand awareness.

SEMYON E. KREWER

Point Lookout, New York

# Introduction

Our hands, together with our eyes, are our most prized possessions. They caress lovingly. They write and they use fork and knife. We rapidly and precisely hit the piano keys with nimble fingers—and we tightly hold a key to turn it to open a door, or a hammer to forcefully drive a nail into the wall. Much of our young life is spent in acquiring manual skills to accomplish these things—training our flexibility, strength, and coordination.

When we contract arthritis, it shows up most of the time first in our hands. Rheumatoid arthritis cripples the fingers so that we are ashamed to show them and they become useless for many tasks. Osteoarthritis, which sooner or later befalls us all, produces knobby finger joints, limiting our motion. Strong pain limits our functioning and threatens our living independently. This is a desolate picture, but there is new hope. If we become aware of all new treatment procedures, medications, heat, splints, and—most importantly—exercise, and know how to protect our hands from damage due to overly strong use, there is hope of avoiding needless crippling.

In this book, I will describe a variety of methods to help your hands and I will outline the usual drug regimen that is prescribed. This will make you more knowledgeable when you talk to your doctor. I will also share with you what I learned about the history of some of these drugs, which I find quite interesting. The main thrust of the book, however, is on physical procedures: exercises, splints, use of heat and cold, proper mix of rest and activity. These are based on my own experience, utilizing some advanced techniques. If you have the help of an occupational/physical therapist, he or she will assist you in choosing from the many self-help devices which I am describing.

Do not consider this book a substitute for seeing a physical therapist, if you are able to see one. In addition to teaching you exercises, the book is meant to make you more knowledgeable about your hands and about physical therapy so that you will be able to converse more accurately with your physician. The more knowledgeable you are, the more fruitful the relationship with your physician will be. Many times I have encountered a harried physician using a vocabulary not normally known to patients. That is why, in this book, I try to familiarize you with this vocabulary concerning joints and muscles. Once you learn it, it takes you less time to communicate. If you do see a physical therapist, that person should evaluate your ranges of motion, train you in carrying out exercises, and encourage you to do them daily. I have heard a lot about "compliance" in connection with exercises. I think the motivation should come out of your own awareness—not from expected punishment or praise by your therapist.

After many years of living with arthritis, I have found that the best way to strike back at this disease is to exercise regularly. But in advocating exercise, I add these important cautions:

1. Do not overexercise. Do the five-minute workout with the Hand Gym once or twice a day for a few months and, after that, once or twice a week to maintain optimum function.
2. Do not neglect your medical routine.
3. Follow rest schedules.
4. Never exercise until painful unless under the advice of a physician.

A five-minute daily workout with the Hand Gym, designed to increase or maintain flexibility and strength of hand muscles and improve hand function, is described. All hand muscles are individually trained with brief isometric exercises. The small (intrinsic) muscles of the hand are stretched to counteract crippling. These exercises have been clinically tested, reported in medical literature, and presented at national and international rehabilitation and rheumatological conferences.

Hints and aids for independent living are presented with extensive descriptions and illustrations of the aids.

The reader will also be acquainted with what can be expected from surgery. This will prepare him better for questions to ask if he is referred to a hand surgeon.

# PART I

Includes many topics that concern arthritics, among them: how the hand functions, the rationale for the exercises, some details about the arthritic disease process, and a discussion of pain and how to deal with it.

All this helpful information will provide both a motivation and a basis for carrying out the exercises that form Part II of this book. You do not have to read all of Part I in order to do the exercises in Part II. Each chapter stands on its own and does not require reading of any other chapter of the book.

I suggest that you scan the topics in Part I and browse in them from time to time; skip any part that may seem too technical for you. The sooner you get to the exercises in Part II, the better.

## THE CHAPTERS

# 1

# Mobilizing to Fight Arthritis

Here in Part I, I want to prepare my readers for the hand exercise system that follows in Part II and, in addition, to discuss a well-rounded program for managing arthritis and for living productively despite the presence of the disease.

## MY EXPERIENCE WITH ARTHRITIS

Although I was in treatment from the start with my rheumatoid arthritis, it was four years before I began working with a physical therapist, and then only because I had developed a hand exercise program (described later) that was of interest to the profession. True, my rheumatologist gave me various sheets with descriptions (but no illustrations) of exercises which I was supposed to perform faithfully. I found these descriptions too abbreviated, and the reasons for doing them were not made clear—moreover, they were simply too strenuous to carry out.

## TYPES OF ARTHRITIS

It will help you to know what type of arthritis you have in order to plan the proper strategy to combat it. You have to rely on your physician for a correct diagnosis.

There are a hundred forms of this disease. The most prevalent are osteoarthritis (noninflammatory) and rheumatoid arthritis, the big crippler (inflammatory). I will present here a very abridged description of the timetables in the disease process and the corresponding disabilities. If you are in treatment, your physician and your therapist will direct you in this matter. The material I am presenting may help you to understand their advice.

## RHEUMATOID ARTHRITIS

As you may know, the progression of rheumatoid arthritis is episodic. The episodes may be as short as a week, or they may go on for a long time. I have suffered episodes lasting more than a year. During an episode you can consider that the disease is *active*. At the end of the episode, the disease becomes inactive and you speak of a *remission*. In some cases the patient may suffer only a single episode with no recurrence. But often the disease flares up again. After a second or third episode, it may then terminate in a remission. If the flare-ups continue to occur over a period of years, the disease finally reaches a chronic stage in which inflammation may or may not be present—but joints have suffered a lot of destruction, and contractures and deformities have set in, possibly to the point where intensive rehabilitation or reconstructive surgery are called for. In my case, the inflammatory process, which is specific for rheumatoid arthritis, was eventually suppressed through gold treatment (monthly injections of a gold solution called myochrysine.)

Typically, during the active phase, I found that one or a few joints, usually the knuckles, became inflamed for limited periods of time, and then the inflammation (redness, heat, and swelling) shifted to other joints. Morning stiffness did not last very long, perhaps less than an hour. Fever was not present, and fatigue was not so great as to prevent near-normal activity.

At some point during the active phase, the sub-acute condition develops into an acute condition. Now the joints become strongly inflamed and the inflammation does not disappear in a few days; fever may be present, and morning stiffness lasts for several hours. Activity is greatly reduced due to fatigue. Although each patient is different, generally the acute phase should not last longer than one or, at most, two weeks if your joints are given a complete rest. Sometimes hospitalization is recommended in severe cases. Usually a variety of anti-inflammatory drugs are given to help bring this acute phase to an end and to reduce the joint inflammation. This is a dangerous time during which much joint destruction is liable to take place. Therefore, joints should be rested completely during this time, and *no active motion exercises should be done*. Isometric exercises are permitted; however, to avoid the danger of adhesions developing near the joint, which would affect elements of the joint such as muscle and capsule tissue and produce severe limitations of joint movement, each joint should be moved passively through the complete range of motion once a day. As the acute phase nears an end, which becomes evident through the fact that all symptoms are lessening, the patient is usually encouraged to do active range-of-motion exercises. The physician makes the important judgment about when to resume a full program of exercises.

In other words, exercises are indicated during all phases of rheumatoid arthritis. During the acute phase, however, motion exercises are passive; that is, they are administered by a therapist or helper to maintain range of motion. The choice and amount of exercises should be discussed with your physician. I describe in this book exercises that are designed to be as pain-free as possible. *If you encounter any pain at all, discuss this with your physician or therapist. Don't try to tough it out.*

## OSTEOARTHRITIS

Osteoarthritis is called the noninflammatory arthritis, although a small amount of heat can be detected over damaged joints, which is indicative of inflammation. (I experienced this with my knees, where a localized area felt warm when I placed my palm over it.) Osteoarthritis is a slowly progressing disease in which the cartilage covering the ends of bones that form the joints is used up and not replaced. One discriminates between *primary* and *secondary* osteoarthritis. Primary osteoarthritis occurs with progressing age. It can start as early as age forty, but the majority of cases seems to occur after age sixty. As the cartilage is depleted, and the joint space thereby reduced, the joint becomes less efficient in function. At first it is uncomfortable and finally it becomes painful. Secondary osteoarthritis is induced either by repetitive trauma (dressmakers and typists often develop arthritic fingers) or by a single trauma to a joint (one patient caught her fingers in a garage door and developed osteoarthritis thereafter). Osteoarthritis resulting from sport injuries may occur at any age. Remember that at age 35 you are more prone to slight injuries of this sort than at 20.

The medications which help most in osteoarthritis are pain killers like aspirin or Tylenol, although the strong anti-inflammatory action of some drugs like Indocin and Clinoril may also be helpful.

## WHERE TO SEEK TREATMENT

Of course, the first move to make when arthritis strikes is to seek sound medical advice. What can we expect from physicians and therapists? In most illnesses, we usually turn to our general practitioner or internist for relief. He or she is most familiar with our lifestyle and medical history and can usually *diagnose* the condition and prescribe the proper treatment. If the treatment does not succeed as expected, we may be sent to consult with a specialist called a *rheumatologist,* who is trained to establish the diagnosis; that is, to tell us which type of arthritis we have, if any. This can be a very complex procedure, requiring many different blood tests, X rays, physical evaluation, and so on. The rheumatologist evaluates these tests and prescribes the proper treatment.

If you have osteoarthritis, most probably you won't need continued treatment by a rheumatologist. He usually reports back to the general practitioner with the diagnosis and recommendation for treatment, which will probably include pain-relieving medication and exercises, as well as other physical therapy modalities.

In the case of *gout,* another form of arthritis, you will probably come under the definitive regimen of medication and diet which helps this condition considerably; it can usually be supervised adequately by the general practitioner.

*Arthritis caused by infection* may be treated with antibiotics and often completely cured. This was the experience of a relative of mine who developed a serious inflammation of her osteoarthritic knees, due to hepatitis. The symptoms disappeared when the hepatitis was overcome.

There are many additional conditions, some highly complex, which can produce arthritic symptoms. One of these is the disease *lupus erythematosus,* which requires close supervision by a specialist. In my case, many tests were performed before lupus could be eliminated as the cause of my arthritic complaints.

*Psoriasis,* too, is often accompanied by arthritic symptoms. I have seen finger joints and knees involved due to psoriasis.

Establishing the diagnosis of rheumatoid arthritis may take time. When my medical diagnosis was finally established, it was two years after the onset of the disease. When I expressed my happiness to my rheumatologist, he was very surprised. "What are you so happy about?" he asked. I answered, "Now that we know what it is, we can fight it." He grinned and replied, "You have a rocky road ahead!" And he was right. We would both have preferred one of the types of arthritis that have a clear-cut, definitive treatment method and can be expected to subside. But I am an optimist by nature, and have faithfully followed all the recommendations of my doctor—even those that tested my resourcefulness, like having to use splints. Finding a hospital where they could be made was something of a research project.

The point here is that *it is extremely important to establish a correct diagnosis of the type of arthritis present.* Only then can you and your doctors chart the proper course of action.

If you want to inform yourself fully about the many types of arthritis, you can request literature from the Arthritis Foundation. There are also quite a few fine books written by physicians on the subject.

The *physiatrist* is a physician who specializes in physical medicine and rehabilitation, and who knows a great deal about kinesiology and exercise. We may be referred to him by the general practitioner, internist, or rheumatologist. He is experienced in understanding the various sources of pain and deformity, and in choosing the treatment modalities that will be most helpful in alleviating pain and improving our ability to function. The array of techniques includes exercise, various heat applications (hot packs, ultrasound, etc.), transcutaneous nerve stimulation (TNS), deep relaxation, and possibly acupuncture at the chronic stage.

Your physiatrist may assign you to a *physical therapist* or an *occupational therapist* or both, and prescribe various forms of treatment. In the early years of arthritis, these professionals are supposed to help you set up your home maintenance program if you are not able to do this by yourself. After later follow-ups, the physiatrist may prescribe splints for individual joints; these will be individually fitted by an occupational therapist.

In the later years of the arthritis, the physical therapist administers therapeutic exercise several times a week to correct deformities; he or she may also administer hot packs and ultrasound treatment, and help with the fitting of canes or walkers, if necessary. The occupational therapist, in later years, may advise you about how to select a wheelchair and suggest adaptive devices for the bathroom and the kitchen that are designed to make daily living easier.

If your pain cannot be managed—i.e., it is intractable and interferes seriously with your functioning—you may be referred to an orthopedic surgeon or hand surgeon.

You may ask, "What remains for the rheumatologist to do?" Plenty. Apart from being in charge of your pharmaceutical regimen, which is a balancing act between drugs and the side effects they produce on your body, he or she will perform general medical checkups to observe your total health picture. Rheumatoid arthritis can attack, directly or indirectly, any organ of the body—directly, by invading organs with the disease; indirectly, through the various side effects of medications (for example, aspirin on the stomach and cortisone on both the stomach and heart). The rheumatologist also ascertains whether any pains in the body are due to diseases other than arthritis. The rheumatologist also tries to consult with you on a balanced lifestyle and the work you can do within the limits of your joint range, just as a doctor advises a cardiac patient to live within the limits of his heart capacity. Thus, we see, the responsibility of the rheumatologist is very great.

I have found all the physicians who have ever helped me with my arthritis to be very concerned people. They have tried to give me the benefit of their experience with the many, many patients they have observed. It has been said of arthritis that no two cases are alike. The severity of the disease and the length of time it lasts are different for all arthritics. It follows, then, that physicians' opinions about the best treatment schedule may vary widely. Rely on your rheumatologist, or—if you are a patient at an arthritis clinic where you are seen by various physicians—rely on the consensus they form about your case. Don't be upset by a divergence of medical opinion. Remember that you, the patient, are the only real judge of whether you are doing better or not. This so-called self-assessment is a very important feedback for the physician or the clinic staff with whom you will chart your future course.

Rheumatoid arthritis, as I have said, is a disease of ups and downs, of flare-ups and remissions. Some lucky people have only one or two flare-ups followed by complete remissions. Most of us, however, continue with the ups and downs. We have remissions between flare-ups, but the remissions are not complete; with each one the joints are further damaged, muscles are weakened, and function is reduced. My rheumatologist described my case as a continuous, slowly smoldering process, with tissue destruction continuing at a slow rate. Now, in the chronic stage, I am mainly concerned with keeping my body as fit as possible and not succumbing to inertia, which undoubtedly would make me an invalid.

## SEEK OUT THE RIGHT HELP

We have to remain optimistic. For all of us, at every stage of the disease, something medical and physical can be done to help. It is up to us, however, to scramble for the right help. Medicine is a very, very wide field, and no physician can be expected to know and be able to carry out all the possible procedures. But our chief attending physician should be able to refer us to the appropriate specialists—the orthopedic surgeon, the physiatrist, the physical or occupational therapist whose particular skills can help us. The Arthritis Foundation supplies names of physicians who specialize in treatment of arthritic patients. These are mostly rheumatologists, but in some regions the lists also contain names of general practitioners, orthopedic surgeons, and physiatrists. The Arthritis Foundation can also furnish the names of rehabilitation institutions, arthritis clinics, hospitals in your area that have occupational and physical therapy departments. To obtain outpatient treatment in these places, referral by your personal physician usually is required.

## THE LESS STRESS THE BETTER

Physicians agree that it is particularly important for arthritics to maintain good health, to avoid colds as much as possible, and to reduce the stresses of life. The general reserve of strength in rheumatoid arthritis is so reduced that any additional strain or stress takes a disproportionate toll. We may have to accept, either by choice or necessity, a cutback of our normal level of work. Trying to do our accusomted work in spite of reduced strength may provoke a flare-up.

The stresses to be avoided include mental or emotional ones, which are known to be a contributing factor to the onset of arthritis as well as to the occurrence of flare-ups. I was told by one physician in charge of a hospital ward for rheumatoid arthritics that on Mondays, following the excitement of Sunday visits by relatives, many patients felt worse.

Direct stresses on the body, such as the climatic stress of cold or humid weather, or a drop in barometric pressure, seem especially stressful for arthritics. To counteract such stresses, we try to wear appropriate clothing and keep our homes comfortable and free of drafts. Some people even spend winters in the sun belt to remain in a favorable climate throughout the year.

Another type of stress on the body is the lack of proper nutrition which can result in poor bowel functions and symptoms of iron and/or vitamin deficiency.

## THE KEY IS PROPHYLAXIS

Although we cannot cure our arthritis, there is much we can do to help ourselves where stress is concerned. Here I come to that large field called "prophylaxis" in rheumatoid arthritis, which is largely the subject of this book. Exercise is one of the most helpful and least utilized techniques of prophylaxis.

I knew little about arthritis in my younger days, but an accident that occurred to a close relative taught me something about osteoarthritis. While playing a game at school she injured her kneecaps, which then started to deteriorate. Her experience demonstrated how an eroded and badly aligned joint becomes susceptible to colds, hepatitis, and other ills. Once I contracted rheumatoid arthritis I realized that I must be kind to my joints, keep them free of stress, and prevent, if possible, infections that might settle in them. This, the first step in the process of "babying oneself," is one of the main prophylactic measures we can use to help deflect the course of the disease.

I have learned, furthermore, that one can relieve the inflammation of the joints through complete rest. Now, after experiencing the use of the hand-rest splints, I understand why: wearing hand-rest splints throughout the night helped considerably to reduce the swelling of my finger joints. If hand-rest splints are not worn during the night the assumption would be that one's hand would still be rested. Apparently, however, the degree of rest they receive is not sufficient; the slightest movement of the hands and fingers during sleep seems to impede the process of reducing inflammation. Similarly for larger joints, you get more benefit from resting comfortably in bed, with a minimum of tossing and turning, than from sitting in a chair and moving only slightly.

Another prophylactic measure is to use an inflamed joint only as much as you can without aggravating it. Let me give you an example. Cortisone injections quickly rid my finger joints of inflammation and pain. But after I wrote two pages in longhand, the inflammation recurred and I had to see my rheumatologist for another injection. The lesson to be learned from this is that we have to find the level at which we can use our joints without aggravating their condition and bringing on inflammation. The judgment can come only from your personal observation, because the degree of one's susceptibility to inflammation is directly related to the severity of the disease, and this changes from time to time.

We can expect our physicians to prescribe drugs to reduce inflammation and suppress the disease to the extent possible, but we can also help ourselves by using the prophylactic means that are available to reduce inflammation. And, most important, we can strive to keep our limbs and body flexible and the muscles as strong and efficient as possible, so as to prevent crippling and loss of function. For most of us, the chances of succeeding in this are excellent. I have found that strong determination and insight is necessary if we are to do the required exercises and to use the other modalities.

There is always a danger that someone reading about the conditions of serious arthritis will become alarmed and discouraged. That is why I like to put the emphasis on prophylaxis—changes in lifestyle, prudence in expending one's energy, daily exercise (very brief sessions), and developing an understanding of how the body works so that we can make intelligent use of splints and other devices and monitor our bodily functions.

## THE STRATEGY FOR FATIGUE

From the onset of my arthritis, I found that after two hours of my normal activities I became so fatigued that I had to rest. Complete rest, preferably in bed, for an hour or two, resulted in more energy for my next back-to-work session of two hours. Sitting in a chair, perhaps reading a book, is *not* a complete rest. Remarkably with relatively little effort we can take care of our daily needs. One-third to one-quarter of the normal strength seems quite all right for me, as long as I retain flexibility. I have learned, however, that in order to maintain even this reduced strength, I require a once-a-week isometric strengthening workout of my muscles; it takes only a few minutes a day for various muscle groups, if spread out over a whole week.

Obviously we want to take the least amount of time out of

our day for rehabilitation—for exercise, hot packs, and so forth. This is what this book is all about. If you allot five to ten minutes in the morning and a short period in the evening for exercises that are not overly strenuous, you give yourself the best chance of being able to continue your normal, useful activities.

## BALANCING REST AND ACTIVITY

Judging the proper mix of rest and activity is crucial. I would like to illuminate this matter in a basic way so that you will be able to figure out, at any one time, whether to rest or to be active.

I suggest this formula for a proper mix:

1. Allot the necessary time for exercise so that the body will be sufficiently strong and flexible to maintain activity.
2. Allow for time in bed—sleeping and resting with the least possible aggravation of the joints.
3. Use the remaining time for the activities of daily living: household chores, work, entertainment, and so forth.

This means that we have to experiment and discover for ourselves how much time we can sneak away for the fruitful activities that make life useful and happy.

# 2
# My Experience with Arthritis Drugs

Note: Let me stress here that I am describing my individual experience with drugs. Please realize that no two cases of arthritis are completely alike and no two patients will react exactly the same way to the same drug.

Arthritis is a chronic disease and after many years of using the same type of drugs some side effects are liable to occur. Therefore, whatever relief can be achieved through physical therapy, exercises, heat and splints is worthwhile trying. However, some people can take aspirin or some of the new nonsteroidal, anti-inflammatory drugs and get benefits from these drugs for many years without side effects. A certain percentage of patients are not helped as much by gold or develop side effects contrary to my experience.

This subject is usually discussed between the doctor and the patient. Arthritis being a chronic disease involving need for pain relief, selection of the most effective drug and consideration of side effects is important. During my seventeen years with arthritis, medications had to be changed a good number of times, due to side effects experienced or loss of effectiveness of some medications that control inflammation and pain.

I feel tempted to describe the drugs in the sequence in which they were prescribed for me, together with my experiences. Please do not feel that you should have been prescribed the same sequence and the same drugs. No two cases are alike.

## BUTAZOLIDIN

During the severe and sudden onset of pain and inflammation (heat, redness, swelling) in my thumb joints and others, I was given Butazolidin three to four times a day. After four days, the inflammation subsided. Butazolidin is one of the most powerful quick-acting anti-inflammation drugs. It can have fairly serious side effects, especially when taken longer than a few days. It can destroy various types of blood cells, resulting in a dangerous anemia as well as in stomach problems. I never met anybody who was prescribed Butazolidin for a prolonged period; but several of my family and friends were prescribed it for inflammatory conditions which could be expected not to last long, such as bursitis of the shoulder. This drug is commonly given to racehorses, I found out, and is known as "Bute." It is supposed to counteract the inflammation that develops during overexertion of the horses' thin sensitive knees, which swell during a race. No explanation as to why this medication works is available.

## ASPIRIN—THE BASIC ARTHRITIS DRUG

The next medication I was told to take as a pain killer was aspirin.

I think it is worthwhile to tell you a little bit about the history of aspirin, the oldest and still most widely used medication for arthritis. Butazolidin has been available only for the last thirty years. It was developed by a Swiss pharmaceutical concern.

The active ingredient of aspirin, salicylic acid, had been known for its medicinal effects already by Hippocrates 2,400 years ago. There are biblical references to it. The North American Indian used infusions of willow bark, which is known to contain salicylate for medicinal purposes. What is the medicinal action of salicylic acid?

1) Pain relieving (analgesic)
2) Fever reducing (antipyretic)
3) Anti-inflammatory (reduces heat, redness, swelling)

About 100 years ago salicylic acid was synthesized. Then Mr. Felix Hoffman, a chemist at the Bayer Co. in Germany developed acetyl salicylic acid in the hope that this compound would be less abrasive to the stomach than salicylic acid. He produced this compound to help his father who suffered from rheumatoid arthritis. So, aspirin was born.

Under the influence of heat and humidity, aspirin (acetyl salicylic acid) can decompose into acetic acid and salicylic acid. You can smell it if you open the bottle, a strong vinegarlike smell. If this is the case, throw the tablets out. Remember that salicylic acid is so strong, it softens corns and callouses.

At first the recommended dose was simply as many as was needed, up to two 5-grain tablets three times a day. I remember my father reminiscing that he imported aspirin from Germany around 1900, when it first became available, to his pharmacy in Moscow. It created a stir among the Russian physicians and was considered a wonder drug. My father reported that physicians prescribed half-tablets to preserve the precious rare supply. I tried the same, using one instead of two tablets at a time. It seemed to work just as well as the larger dose; that is, only in a limited way, some individual finger joints remained very painful. After rheumatoid arthritis was finally diagnosed by my rheumatologist, he increased my dose to three tablets four times a day. This was supposed to increase the salicylate level in my blood to counter inflammation, and thereby produce pain killing in addition to the direct pain killing action of aspirin on brain centers. He warned me to be on the lookout for ringing in the ears (effect on the brain) or upset stomach, which are side effects to be expected. For about three and a half years I was on this regimen. I was more comfortable, less stiff with this high dose of aspirin, but some large and small knuckles of both hands were always red, especially in winter, and were very painful when using the hands.

I had to stop taking aspirin when my stomach started to become very painful and bloated. It started with hyperacidity. Taking antacids, using buffered aspirins (Bufferin), and even Ecotrin (coated aspirin that dissolves further down the gastrointestinal tract, beyond the stomach) did not help. The salicylates find their way to the stomach walls through the blood, if not directly by way of mouth, and do their dirty work. Stomach X rays (upper G.I.) did not divulge an ulcer, but some "occult" (hidden) blood was found in the stool. This, I was told, could be expected in most people taking such large doses of aspirin. Keep in mind that the active ingredients in solutions used to soften corns and calluses is salicylate; you can imagine what it could do to your stomach wall. I have not been able to take aspirin since. For many people, however, aspirin is truly the best drug—and can be tolerated.

## NONSTEROIDAL ANTI-INFLAMMATORY DRUGS

Fortunately, some new, so-called nonsteroidal anti-inflammatory drugs came into the market at that time. Steroids (cortisone) are considered too dangerous for a chronic condition because of the variety of side effects. I tried Brufen, which was available in England. This drug is now available here as Motrin (ibuprofen). It worked for me—using one to two tablets a day—for a year with wonderful results, after which it produced strong headaches, even though I reduced the dose to one-quarter of amount prescribed! Then a new nonsteroidal became available in England and Mexico: Naprosyn (now also available in the U.S.). I was careful to take ½ tablet two times per day, which worked very well for me, even beyond the time I started to receive gold treatment. Then I suffered sudden, severe stomach bleeding, without any previous warning of pain, nausea, or other symptoms. Nobody can trace this occurrence to Naprosyn, but my physician stopped me from taking this drug again. I was told that all anti-inflammatory drugs can have a deleterious effect on the stomach.

I took Clinoril for a while which I found very effective, much more so than Indocin, the first nonsteroidal, anti-inflammatory drug. However, stomach symptoms made me discontinue this drug. Many people, however, can take some of these drugs for years without problems.

## CORTISONE

The anti-inflammatory effect of cortisone was discovered in the late 1940s by Dr. P. Hench, who was rewarded with a Nobel Prize for this research. It appeared as a dramatic solution to cure arthritis symptoms, and was hailed as a miracle drug in the wake of the other two miracle drugs—sulfa and penicillin, discovered in the same decade. However, in the course of time, the serious side effects of cortisone were discovered and it is used only very sparingly today.

I received cortisone injections into my finger joints, one at a time, sometimes repeated after a number of weeks. I also received, occasionally, a cortisone injection into a very painful shoulder. During the time I received those injections I did not have to take any aspirin. The cortisone was only partially used up locally and that part which spilled over into the general circulation produced wonders of well-being. Some cortisone, a steroid hormone, is produced daily in the body by the cortex rind of the adrenal glands. The two adrenal glands are endocrine glands which release adrenaline into the bloodstream with the known effect of "revving you up." Cortisone in limited amounts for brief periods seems to be fairly harmless. Concert pianists are known to use it to overcome back pain during long performances. Too many repeated joint injections, however, seem to practically "dissolve away" some tissues, leaving the joints thin and unstable. Larger amounts by repeated administration in form of tablets may result in stomach problems (including ulcers) and increased blood pressure. Continued use can also cause weakening of bones by calcium loss, and even cataracts. I had to drop cortisone after about nine months. The actress, Rosalind Russell, apparently took small amounts of cortisone for many years.

## GOLD AND PENICILLAMINE

The beneficial effect of gold was discovered accidentally by a French father and son physician team by the name of Forestier in the 1920s. The Forestiers were physicians at a spa in France where they saw many arthritics. The young Forestier suffered from tuberculosis with strong arthritic symptoms in some joints. The Forestiers tried to treat the tuberculosis, for which there was no cure available at that time other than fresh mountain air, with gold salts. It was *en vogue* at that time to use heavy metals for various disease conditions; lead had been very successful with certain diseases. After administration of gold, young Forestier's arthritic symptoms disappeared, but not the tuberculosis. They then tried gold on arthritic patients in their spa with success.

I was finally placed on a gold regimen which involved many weeks of solganol (waxy) or myochrisine (watery solution) gold injections. Blood and urine tests were carried out at first before each injection. Gold can be toxic to many patients. It can be harmful to the kidneys and destroy blood cells. It can also produce a rash which, if gold is not discontinued, can cover the whole body and cause death. In fact, I did not agree to gold treatment for several years as one of my attending physicians had witnessed such a death of a patient on gold through so-called defoliation and warned me against its use. After an initial period of accumulating sufficient gold in the body, I now receive gold injections once a month. Urine and blood tests are done four times a year. Whereas most physicians have experience in administering and checking for side effects of most drugs used to treat arthritis, this is not the case for gold, due to the seriousness of side effects and the complicated regimen. I notice this when I am away from my home base for extended periods of time. I have with me always a letter from my rheumatologist, outlining my gold regimen and confirming that I have never had any side effects. Still, I have difficulties finding a physician willing to administer the gold shots, even though I carry the vial of Solganol or Myochrysine with me. Several times, I have had to go to a hospital which has a "gold clinic," be interviewed by a local rheumatologist, and have blood and urine evaluation to finally receive the gold shot. It is a very inconvenient procedure, but very much worth my while. Gold in the form of tablets has been promised for the last five years and should be available soon. Unfortunately, gold does not "work" (i.e. suppress inflammation) for everybody.

A new drug, penicillamine, has become available in the last few years. It has been tested cooperatively here and in Russia. The inflammation-suppressing qualities and side effects are reported to be similar to those of gold. At this time, probably fewer physicians are familiar with the regimen for penicillamine than for gold. There are also some symptoms which are not suppressed. When the weather changes, and/or I use some joints beyond my limits, I have some involvements. Therefore, I have been prescribed Clinoril as an auxiliary nonsteroid anti-inflammatory drug. I developed stomach symptoms after two months of using Clinoril and restrict it now to occasional use or take Tylenol (acetaminophen), which is a pain killer but not an anti-inflammatory drug. Many people, however, are greatly helped by Clinoril without severe side effect symptoms.

In osteoarthritis Tylenol and any of the nonsteroidal anti-inflammatory drugs are used. One of the first (and cheapest) of the latter is Indocin, which never worked for me, but is reported effective in osteoarthritis.

## CODEINE AND TYLENOL

Another drug with a very powerful pain killer, but with no anti-inflammatory action, is codeine. It is a narcotic, and can therefore cause addiction, so is not prescribed for chronic conditions. It is available by itself or in combination with aspirin or now even with Tylenol. I was once prescribed codeine during a bout with bursitis of the shoulder. I will never forget the sweet warmth penetrating my shoulder, arm, and body, permitting much needed sleep. I then realized the addictive qualities of narcotics. Beware! Tylenol is an effective replacement for aspirin as a pain killer, has no bad effect on the stomach, but lacks anti-inflammatory properties. It is a poor substitute for aspirin in rheumatoid arthritis where inflammation has to be fought in addition to pain.

## LINIMENTS AND RUBS

From this odyssey of drug experiences it is quite evident that whatever benefit you can receive from nondrug, non–side-effect physical therapy, exercises, splints, and heat is a specially precious adjunct. Liniments and rubs externally applied can be quite helpful for temporary pain relief. Ben-Gay (active ingredient salicylate) or Banalg (active ingredient camphor) extend for quite a while the pleasant effect of a hot whirlpool bath. There are many other liniments and rubs for you to try. I found some of them too harsh for my skin. But they are evidently okay for others, otherwise they would not be advertised and sold.

## DMSO

Now to DMSO and its peculiar story. More than fifteen years ago a worker in a wood pulp plant accidentally poured the industrial solvent DMSO (dimethylsulfoxide) over his painful wrist. The pain vanished. This was reported in the press. Since that time, many books and untold papers and studies have been published on DMSO. To date this substance is federally released only for bladder condition (interstitial cystitis). However, for the longest time DMSO was not accepted for use against arthritis pain. However use of DMSO is generally permitted at the time of this writing for use in Florida, Louisiana, Oklahoma, Washington, Texas, and Oregon

No DMSO of medicinally pure quality is marketed even in these states as yet. A physician in Florida prescribed and furnished me with some DMSO to try for my joints. I applied it after very careful cleaning of the skin (washed several times) to the root of my thumb, my shoulder and elbow, and my knees. I felt some warmth in my thumb and could immediately exercise it through a larger range of motion. This excellent effect lasted several months. The effect on the elbows was less pronounced, on the shoulder minimal, on the knee zero. Once when I applied DMSO (75% solution) to the thumbs, I had not washed my hands thoroughly before. The same day I experienced some influenza-like pain in my legs and arms. This condition, not accompanied by any head cold symptoms, I figured, could have come about through some toxic substance on the skin, which may have penetrated into the bloodstream, carried in by the

DMSO. I had read that DMSO is a "penetrant" which can, for instance, take DDT into the bloodstream. Try to obtain a *medicinally* pure 75% solution of DMSO. A 99.9% pure *solvent* obtained from a paint store contains a 0.1% impurity which may penetrate into your bloodstream with unforeseeable effects. Once DMSO is released, proper precaution for its use will be published. Most, but not all, people using DMSO develop a strong garlic- or oyster-type mouth odor. I was lucky—I experienced hardly any odor, perhaps due to the fact that I applied DMSO very sparingly by means of an eye dropper. A more liberal application of the drug is indicated on the large joints. I experienced some slight temporary painful skin rash after the first application on each area. No DMSO of medicinally pure quality is marketed as yet even in those states in which its use is permitted.

## TRANQUILIZERS

Two mg. Valium, twice a day, was prescribed for me by my rheumatologist to help counteract muscle stiffness. I took it religiously for a long period until I developed severe mental problems with self identity which I attributed to the Valium. Withdrawal side effects were very disagreeable for two days. After that I was the "normal" arthritic again.

## VITAMIN C AND FLU VACCINATIONS

500 mg. per day was prescribed to me by my rheumatologist. It seems that vitamin C is conducive to keeping joint tissues in shape. Furthermore, anything which *might* prevent colds is important for the arthritic. Yearly flu shots are an additional helpful preventive measure.

Note again that all the above represents my personal experience which cannot be expected to apply directly to your condition.

More complete information on arthritis drugs is available from the Arthritis Foundation.

# TABLE OF DRUGS

**Analgesic (painkiller) not anti-inflammatory**

Tylenol
Codeine (careful!)

**Anti-inflammatory**

Butazolidin (short use only)
Cortisone (tablets and injections)

**Analgesic, nonsteroidal, anti-inflammatory**

Aspirin
Indocin (relatively cheap)
Motrin
Naprosyn
Nalfon*
Clinoril
Tolectin*
More can be expected in the future

**Gold preparations, inflammation suppressants**

Solganol
Myochrysine
Penicillaminc*

**Liniments, Rubs**

Ben-Gay (basic active ingredient, salicylate)
Banalg (basic active ingredient, camphor)
DMSO (check whether its use is allowed in your state; follow your doctor's recommendations)

**General Supportive Medications**

Valium (tranquilizer to help stiffness; I had bad side effects)
Yearly flu shots (important!)
Vitamin C

* No personal experience

# 3
# Body Mechanics

If the human body came with an owner's manual, complete with a parts list and repair hints, many of our health problems could be solved easily. But this is not the case. The body is a mystery to most of us, despite what we learn about it in health and biology classes at school. Not even a physician can be expected to know everything about the body, its malfunctioning, and repair. That is why there are so many specialists in medicine who concern themselves with a limited aspect of the body and its malfunctioning.

If we have arthritis, it is important to increase our knowledge of the body. We are concerned with the functioning of the whole body—not only the skeleton and muscles and ligaments, but also the temperature, circulation, breathing, and some aspects of the nervous system. Increased knowledge will help us to observe our condition and describe it to our physician and, most importantly, will enable us to understand the reasons for the prophylactic measures that are recommended to us, especially exercises.

## OUR MARVELOUS BODY RESOURCES

Essentially the human is an ''animal'' that moves about and adapts itself to needs. When the body is not sufficiently used, it loses the capacity to make the most of its possibilities: bones and teeth decalcify if not used; muscles become flabby and weak when they are not regularly exercised. On the other hand, if demand on the body increases, we have a remarkable capacity to adapt ourselves: when called upon to function, muscles can increase in bulk, and bones and ligaments can become stronger. The healthy body also can adapt to hot and cold climates, to high and low humidity, and to varying air pressure. The healthy body, furthermore, has a remarkable capacity for self-repair. A cut in the skin will heal by itself, and a broken bone, when properly set, will become as strong as before.

Both adaptability and self-repair are somewhat limited in arthritics. They can never develop the muscle bulk of the bodybuilder, for instance, since their damaged joints prevent the muscles from being exercised to their limit. In arthritis, also, there is a lessening of adaptability to climatic changes, especially to cold, humidity, and changes in air pressure. As far as self-repair is concerned, it no longer holds true for the joint structures. Cartilage, once used up, is not replaced. Ligaments, once stretched, do not regain their original elasticity.

Arthritics, then, have to follow a narrow, prophylactic path. We have to avoid the excesses to which we cannot adapt ourselves as easily as before. We have to prevent as much damage as possible in order to reduce the need for repair.

## THE EXERCISER'S VOCABULARY

I will start the discussion with some nomenclature of interest to arthritics, including words used in anatomy to describe directions and locations of certain parts of the body. This will help you to converse better with your physician and therapist.

*Anterior* denotes everything located on the front part of the body; *posterior* anything on the back of the body. Moving the extremities laterally (to the side, away from the center line of the body) is called *abduction*. Moving the extremities medially (toward the center line of the body) is called *adduction*.

When referring to hands, abduction means moving the fingers away from the middle line (the middle finger) and adduction means moving them toward the middle line.

The word *proximal* (in proximity) means a position closer to the body; the word *distal* (more distant), a position farther away from the body. For example, if you look at a diagram of a skeleton you will note that the femur bone is proximal to the knee joint, and the tibia and fibula are distal to the knee joint.

In general, to *extend* a joint means to hold it straight; to *flex* it means to exert muscle power to bend the joint. However, there is no definitive direction for *flexion*.

When we talk about the *phalanges* of the hands and feet, we talk about the fingertips as the *distal phalanges;* they are farthest from the body. The *proximal phalanges* are the bones of the fingers or toes that are attached to the main part of the hand or foot; the bones between the proximal and the distal phalanges are the *middle phalanges*.

Individual bones form *joints* with neighboring bones. These joints, most of which are flexible, are often formed so that the head of the distal bone fits into the base of the proximal bone. The head is often spherical, fitting the base of the adjoining bone in a way that permits both bones to rotate in several directions. An example of a ball-and-socket joint is the hip. The spherical head of the femur fits into its corresponding firm base, called the acetabulum, in the pelvis.

Many joints are far more complicated than this, however. In the wrist, for example, the ulna of the forearm articulates (contacts and rotates) against various carpal bones. The shoulder is another complex joint.

There is usually a lining of cartilage on the ends of the bones to facilitate smooth gliding of the joint. An X ray of a joint shows what is called joint space—a narrow space separating the cartilaginous ends of the bones. If the cartilage is used up and is not replaced, as in osteoarthritis, or if it is eroded, as in rheumatoid arthritis, the ends of the bones come closer together and one talks about a reduced joint space.

The membrane that defines and encloses the joint space is called the *synovium* (figure 1); the synovial fluid it secretes lubricates the joint. In rheumatoid arthritis this thin inner skin swells and becomes inflamed. The inflammation in turn may cause the capsule of the joint to become distended. The capsule, which surrounds the joint, may consist of ligaments, muscle fibers, and other connective tissue. *The pain in arthritis is mostly due to the stretching and twisting of the ligaments and capsules.*

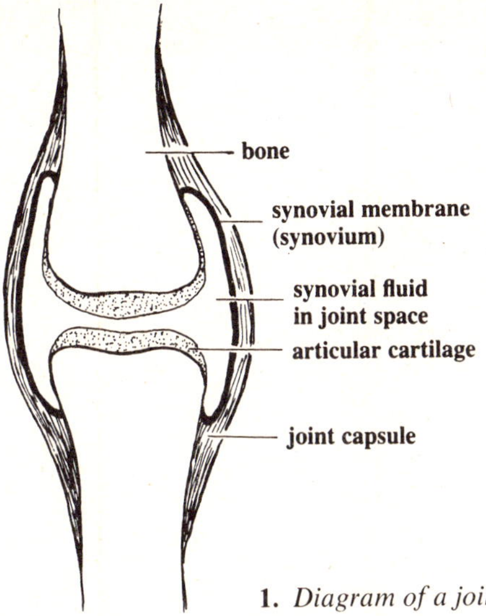


1. *Diagram of a joint*

## VULNERABLE JOINTS IN ARTHRITIS

It will be helpful to study the following drawings of the hand to familiarize yourself with the anatomical names of the various bones and joints (figures 2 and 3). Occupational therapists who

2. *Anatomical names for joints and bones of the hands*

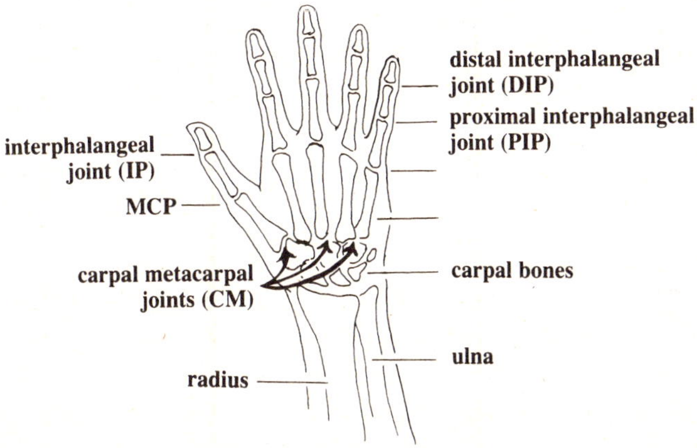

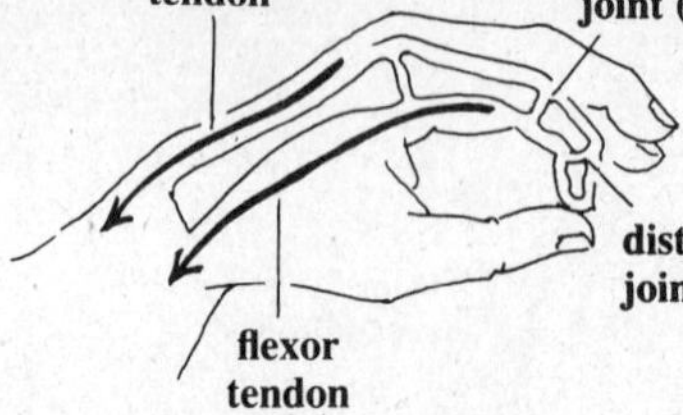


**3.** *Function of hand joints when grasping an object between the tip of the finger and the thumb*

deal with arthritics try to teach these terms to their patients to facilitate communication about bones, joints, deformities, protective positions, exercise positions, and so forth.

A few joints, such as the distal interphalangeal joints of the fingers, are predisposed to osteoarthritis. The joints that are mostly involved in rheumatoid arthritis are the proximal interphalangeal joints and the metacarpal phalangeal joints (big knuckles). In the acute phase of the disease inflammation can be expected in several of the big knuckles. The corresponding joints in the feet, the metatarsal phalangeal joints, are often similarly involved.

Frequently in rheumatoid arthritis the symmetrical joints—the same joints on either side of the body—are involved simultaneously. In osteoarthritis the involvement is more often one-sided, possibly due to increased stress on a single joint.

In the later stages of rheumatoid arthritis, osteoarthritis is superimposed. Whether rheumatoid arthritis or osteoarthritis, the same types of exercises and physical treatment are indicated. Shortening of the range of motion and weakening of the muscles around the joint are common complaints in both types of arthritis.

## WHICH TYPE OF ARTHRITIS?

X rays form only one part of the diagnostic criteria (established by a conference of international rheumatism associations) used in rheumatoid arthritis. Other criteria taken into account include swelling and redness of joints, sedimentation rate, and other blood tests such as hemoglobin, fatigue, morning stiffness, reduction of range of motion of various joints, reduced strength of hand grip, and functional complaints. A certain percentage of the criteria has to be positive over a certain length of time in order to confirm the diagnosis of rheumatoid arthritis.

Osteoarthritis will show a different X ray profile, mainly reduction of joint space. This indicates decreased cartilage.

## THE MUSCLES

The muscles that move the bones are called *skeletal muscles*. They originate on a proximal bone and are usually inserted into a distal bone, which is moved by the muscle tendon. Figure 4 shows how muscles connected to a set of bones are pulling the distal bone into flexion.

The muscle pulling in the desired direction is called the *agonist*. The muscle pulling in the opposite direction is called the *antagonist*. Some muscles are called *synergists;* they aid in completing the desired motion. The antagonist muscles have the important function of stabilizing the joint so that the agonist does not pull it apart. They also hinder the too rapid and forceful contraction of the agonist, especially as the joint action is a learned reflex, information for which is stored in the spinal column. Observe how the toddler walks. He would like to walk in

4. *Skeletal muscle function*

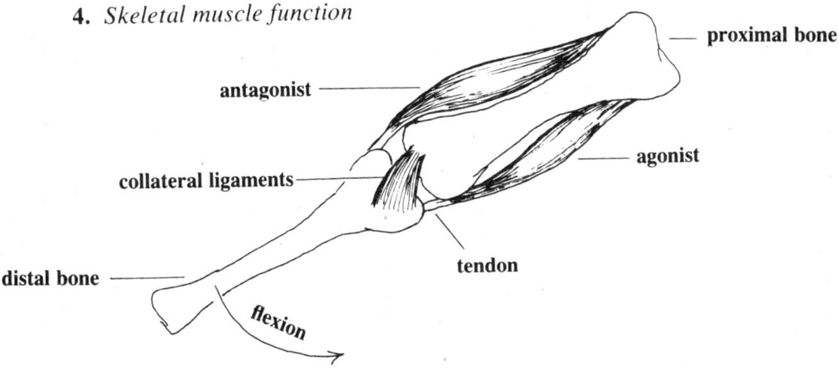

a straight line like the grownup, but he does not quite succeed at first. He *learns* to walk in a straight line. The coordination necessary for this is based on learned reflexes which keep him from overshooting his gait to one side or the other. Walking in a straight line, then, is coordinated through a reflex. That is why sleepwalkers walk straight in their sleep.

## FUNCTIONAL ANATOMY OF THE HAND

The fingers of each hand are moved by thirty-two muscles (figure 5). These are fifteen extrinsic muscles (A, E, F), located in the forearm, and 18 intrinsic small muscles, located within the hand (e,f,a,o). E,e denote extensor muscles; F, f indicate flexor muscles; a denotes abductors and adductors; and o are oppenens muscles which rotate the thumb and the middle finger.

The *extrinsic muscles* are so called because they are located outside the hand. They can be felt in the forearm. The most powerful muscles of this group are the *flexors*. The flexor superficialis (sublimus) lies close to the surface of the underside of the arm and is the most powerful of all the hand muscles. It bends the middle phalanx. When you carry a heavy suitcase or grip a hammer tightly to drive in a nail, this is the muscle doing the work. Behind the superficialis muscle, closer to the bone of the lower arm, is the profundus (deep seated) muscle. This muscle bends the distal phalanx, providing precision gripping or tapping when you hold a pen in writing, or play the piano, or

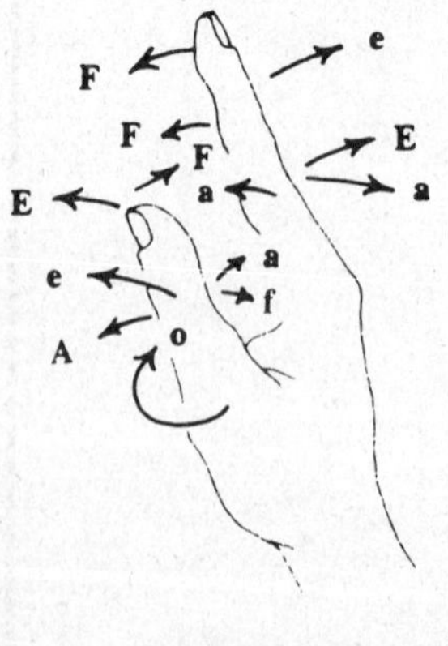


5. *Thirty-two muscles move the fingers of the hand*

use the typewriter. Its antagonist is the small thin and long lumbricalis (rainworm) muscle. Understanding of the function of this muscle has long eluded us and is still controversial. I follow the belief that this muscle acts like a precision brake to control the more powerful extrinsic profundus flexor, thus creating an interplay between these muscles to permit rapid and precise fingering such as when playing trills on a piano.

The extrinsic extensor muscle is located on top of the forearm, extending the MCP joints. It is a very weak antagonist to the powerful flexors. Frequently in rheumatoid arthritis this muscle becomes very weak; its tendons across the MCP joints become dislodged due to the disease, as ligaments and fibers of the capsules become weakened. Ulnar deviation and inability to straighten the hand often result.

Now to the *intrinsic muscles*. They are so called because they are located inside the hand. We already talked about the lumbricalis muscle, which meanders from its origin on the profundus flexor in the palm of the hand to the side of the MCP joints; beyond the joint, at the side of the proximal phalanx, it shoots out its tendon which crawls (just like a rainworm) to the top of the phalanx to cross over the small finger joints and finally insert (end) at the base of the distal phalanx.

The most prominent of the intrinsic muscles are the *interossei,* so called because they are located between the metacarpal bones of the hand. There is one on each side of the long fingers. You can feel the interosseus No. 1 located between the index finger and the thumb. When you pinch you can feel the muscle belly of this muscle get hard. The interossei muscles can move the fingers sideways (abduct and adduct). They can also rotate the fingers. All of them except interosseus No. 1 extend the PIP joints. The two interossei at the sides of each finger can bend the proximal phalanx of that finger.

There are several intrinsic muscles of the thumb. They are all located in what seems like a single large muscle belly at the root of the thumb in the palm, referred to as the thenar eminence. In reality there are several muscles there which abduct, adduct, and flex; one of them, the opponens, rotates the thumb.

On the opposite side of the palm is located the hypothenar eminence, at the foot of the little finger. It covers the muscle bellies of the opponens muscle, which rotates the little finger, and of the small intrinsic flexor, which bends the little finger at the MCP joint.

The multitude of actions by the various intrinsic muscles facilitates the miraculous agility and dexterity of the hand. In rheumatoid arthritis contracture (shortening) of these intrinsic muscles is a typical occurrence and therefore, understandably, interferes seriously with our normal hand function. Exercises to counteract this contracture are therefore very important. Only in recent years has it become clear which positions of the fingers will stretch the intrinsic muscles. See exercises in chapter 6.

## HOW THE WRIST ASSISTS IN HAND FUNCTION

Most of us think of the wrist as a simple joint that permits the hand to move up or down and left or right, or to rotate in reference to the forearm, thereby helping us to reach into various places with our palm and fingers. This is only half the story. The wrist is by no means a simple joint. It is also referred to as the *carpus*. It consists of seven carpal bones arranged in two rows between the metacarpal bones and the radius and the ulna of the forearm. When the wrist moves, the carpal bones mostly glide against each other as well as against the radius and the ulna, in a great variety of directions. All gliding bone surfaces are equipped with a synovium, as are the tendon sheaths surrounding the many extensor tendons on the dorsum (top surface) of the hand. In rheumatoid arthritis any of these synovia and tendon sheaths are liable to get inflamed and painful. The result is that we let the hand drop and do not extend the fingers to avoid pain.

The question arises in what way this limits our function, and here we will describe a very important aspect of how the wrist in its various positions assists the powerful extrinsic finger muscles. You may have noted that when you grip a hammer tightly to drive a nail into the wall, the wrist is automatically bent up. This position gives the powerful flexor muscles a slight stretch to make them operate at highest efficiency. You can feel the slight stretch of those muscles by digging your thumb into the

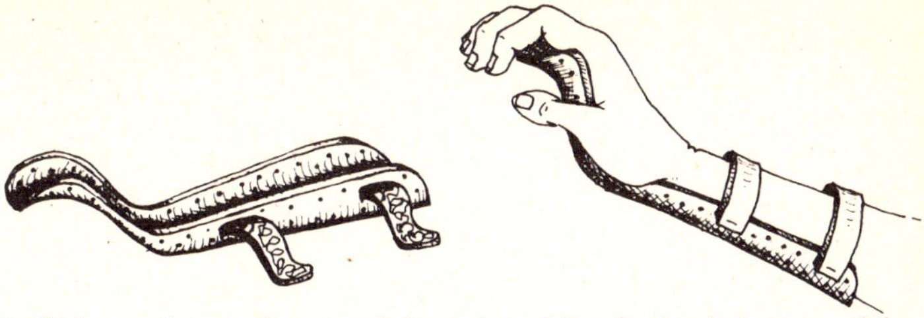

6. *Wrist cock-up splint rests the wrist while placing it in a good functional position.*

muscle belly of the lower arm and moving the wrist of that arm up and down. You will notice that as the wrist is moved up, the muscle belly tightens somewhat. This tightening helps the performance of the flexor muscle.

The performance of the extensor muscle is helped by moving the wrist down. This helps to stretch the extrinsic extensors. In writing, for instance, the wrist is usually held either straight or slightly bent.

If the wrist is inflamed, there is a tendency to drop it down. To counteract this, to avoid stiffening of the wrist in this position and also to help in functioning, I've used a very simple splint which is available from surgical supply stores (figure 6). Called a wrist cock-up splint, it consists of a metal trough into which you fit your underarm; it has a small spoon-like extension that supports your wrist in a good functional position. This splint interferes relatively little with grasping and, at the same time, rests the wrist to prevent pain.

## CIRCULATION AND THE ROLE OF THE LYMPHATIC SYSTEM

In order for the muscles to become warm and to function well, we need increased *circulation.* In the circulatory system, the blood flows out from the aorta through the arteries, the arterioles, and eventually to the smallest of all vessels, the capillaries. The capillaries transport the blood to the individual cells, diffusing oxygen and other necessary supplies to them through microscopic spaces in the capillary walls. In return, waste materials from the cells move into the capillaries, and are carried back in the bloodstream through the venous system to the right atrium of the heart, before going to the lungs. Some of the "waste" carried back through the veins is in the form of carbon dioxide. In the lungs, the carbon dioxide is eliminated from the blood (as in the exhaust of a car) and replaced by oxygen (as in the carburetor) from the air we breathe.

Circulation also means pumping out of the muscle metabolic waste products other than carbon dioxide—for instance lactic acid, which is removed through the lymphatic part of the circulatory system. When lactic acid is left to accumulate in muscles, they become painful and stiff and tend to retain water. Let us find out why this accumulation of metabolic waste takes place, and how we can promote the healthy process of waste removal so as to avoid pain and stiffness. The muscles, as you will see, play a reciprocating role in this process.

The insides of the veins are equipped with little flaps which allow the blood to move in one direction only. The flow is kept up partly due to the pumping action of the heart together with compression of the veins by the muscles (one speaks of the "muscle pump").

The lymphatic system at first appears to be less ingeniously designed. Whereas the capillary endings of the arteries are intermittently intertwined with the corresponding venous capillaries, producing relatively little resistance to the flow of blood between the two systems, the lymphatic vessels collect their liquid and waste rather loosely from all the nooks and crannies of the body and get no push from the arterial system.

The lymphatic system, among its other duties, picks up particles entering the body through the skin that have to be prevented from entering the blood stream lest they cause mechanical obstruction or infection in some of the organs. When someone is bitten by an insect, for example, the lymphatic system sets up a defense. Bacteria and viruses can be deposited in the skin through the insect bite together with solid particles of the insect's stinger. These are picked up by the lymphatic system in a defense network of flexible tubes equipped with flaps similar to those of the veins. The tubes cannot serve every single tiny spot of the skin. Therefore, a small pressure differential (suction) from the distal end of the tubes collects the wastes, including particles and bacteria. If the lymphatic system is unable to collect the bacteria, a localized infection with inflammation is produced; a pimple forms which eventually bursts, thus eliminating some of the waste directly from the body.

A similar process occurs with solid particles too large to be absorbed by the lymphatic system. Think of a wooden splinter. If you permit the skin to heal over the splinter, white blood cells will start to fight against the intruder, as evidenced by pus and swelling. When the splinter is removed, the lymph continues to act to remove any debris and swelling. Waste travels through the tubes to the next lymph node in the network. These nodes are little organs located in places such as the elbow, neck, knee, and groin. Lymphocytes, white blood cells that abound in lymph nodes, fight the intruding particles and sometimes digest them in order to bring them into a shape which will be harmless when they enter the bloodstream. The various lymph tubes collect into larger pipes as they move proximally, and these eventually empty into a large vein. Some poisons, such as rattlesnake venom, may not be stopped at a lymph node; if circulation is not stopped by a tourniquet and the poison sucked out at the point of entry, it may spread throughout the bloodstream and cause severe illness. Some viruses, like that of sleeping sickness, can completely immobilize a lymph node so that no liquid can pass through it, resulting in a swollen arm or leg.

The importance of maintaining good lymphatic circulation is obvious. To keep the lymph flowing, the system relies on the compressing action of the muscles and on the little flap valves within the lymph tubes. In the extremities, circulation of lymph is accomplished by the motion of the arms and legs. In the torso, it is helped along by breathing—namely by the muscle action of the diaphragm, the intercostal muscles, and the various other muscles that expand and contract the rib cage. Some lymph tubes ride piggyback on arteries and benefit from the pulsation of the blood through the arteries. The lymph flow is also increased by stronger blood flow, which can be encouraged by applying heat to the skin or rubbing it with a counterirritant ointment such as Ben-Gay.

If skin temperature is lowered slightly, lymph flow will be decreased near the skin. When a stye—an infection at the root of an eyelash, caused usually by some dust or other particle—forms, you are usually told to apply warm compresses. I have been able to make a stye vanish by applying compresses at the outset. This is due to the speedup of the lymph drainage. Once the stye is in full bloom, however, the warm compresses will still help to open the stye and let the infection drain. This demonstrates the importance of maintaining warm skin temperature to keep the lymph flowing. (Some amphibious animals, like frogs, which spend time submerged in cold water, have special lymph hearts to help them maintain their lymph circulation.)

Fluid from the joints, specifically the joints of hands and feet, also drains through the lymphatic system, passing through delicate passages to the lymph vessels of the skin. It seems to follow from this that elimination of fluid from the joints will be enhanced by increasing circulation in the skin. Hence we arrive at the relevance of this discussion for arthritics. It seems to me very important that we become aware of how our lymphatic system functions, in order to understand better the various physical therapy modalities available for treating our arthritic discomforts.

It is known that in rheumatoid arthritis the circulation becomes sluggish. This is probably due, in part at least, to the fact that arthritics make less use of their muscles; they move about less to avoid joint pain. Since most of the heat of the body is produced within the muscles, the temperature balance in the arthritic shifts somewhat in the direction of decreased surface temperature. (Cold hands and feet are often reported by arthritics. I myself have noticed a feeling of cold around my ankles, knees, and hips. For a while I felt this also on the shoulders, but the discomfort in these joints disappeared after a series of mudpack treatments. I protect my ankles by wearing woollen socks of suitable weight during both summer and winter. I wear woollen knee warmers and woollen underwear or binders to protect flanks and hips. I find that I suffer considerably less pain in these various joints when I cover them with wool.)

Just as it disposes of viruses, bacteria, and particles from the skin, the lymphatic system also removes such items from the joint spaces. Viruses and bacteria may enter the joint space through the bloodstream and the lymph system has to remove them in order to prevent a localized infection and inflammation. The job of the lymph system can be compared to that of a filter in which the undesirable particles are withdrawn from circulation and kept immobolized within the lymph nodes. Solid particles of ground-up cartilage are likely to appear in a joint space; in some cases, the particles may even be bone ground up through the movement of the joint. Once the lymph spaces and channels around a joint are damaged through inflammation, lymph clearance becomes more difficult. At such times, heat and muscle action help to increase the flow of lymph from around the joints, thereby decreasing pressure and pain. I have noticed that very strong heat often has an immediate (but not necessarily permanent) effect in removing pain, particularly in the feet, hands, and hips. The gentle warmth of a heating pad has very little effect. With hands and feet, I have obtained best results by using a whirlpool bath. For the hip, a Hydrocolator pack or, at home, application of a turkish towel dipped into very hot water works best. Gentle heat, on the other hand, is indicated for the lower back, as very strong heat there might irritate nerves which emanate near the vertebrae. I find hot mudpacks, a treatment available at certain spas, to be the best treatment for shoulders and knees. The effect of heat can be prolonged by the application of Ben-Gay or a similar liniment.

Atmospheric pressure also influences the functioning of the lymphatic system. Arthritics generally do not feel well when the barometric pressure decreases, as before a storm. It is noteworthy that increasing the pressure uniformly on the skin, with stretch gloves, for example, makes arthritics feel more comfortable.

## FOR BETTER LYMPHATIC ACTION

A perfect modality to increase lymphatic drainage is the combination of heat and massage in the form of a very warm whirlpool bath. All people get beneficial results from these baths;

arthritics can expect the special benefit of relief from pain. To take full advantage of the massaging action, you may want to maneuver yourself directly into the stream of the jets—but be careful, because the force may be too powerful for comfort. I have found that both the small whirlpool for hands and feet and the unit which is fastened to the tub can be controlled well for my individual needs, regarding temperature as well as strength and direction of the jet.

Lymphatic drainage is important in arthritis not only for the joints, but also for the muscles. If the skin above the muscle cools suddenly, we get a chill in the area which might produce a muscle spasm, such as lumbago in the lower back. But any muscle may be painful when lymphatic drainage does not remove the metabolic waste products of muscle activity. The so-called charley horse is a case of a muscle being overly strained so that the lymph cannot remove the waste quickly enough. In the arthritic, lymph drainage will be sluggish and produce pain or stiffness even with minimal or no use of the muscles. The typical morning stiffness may be at least partially due to the fact that the lymph system is sluggish and requires some additional impetus to increase circulation, like a warm bath and some moving about.

You are aware that when you get up in the morning your feet are usually very slightly swollen. Your walking shoes feel a little tight at first when you put them on. If you use bedroom slippers for a while, the swelling will abate due to the pumping action of the muscles within the legs, which circulates the fluids upward. Don't be surprised if this effect is particularly pronounced in arthritis.

I have gone into some detail regarding possible interconnection between lymphatic function and the symptoms of an arthritic, and the significance these interconnections may have for certain types of physical treatments. I have never come across this subject mentioned in any other book on the subject of arthritis. The reason for this lack, I suspect, is that the lymphatic system is very difficult to monitor. Only recently, with the advent of radioisotope tracing techniques, has it been possible to determine the speed of lymph flow. Slow clearance of lymph from joints of patients with rheumatoid arthritis, as compared

ularly. Physiologically, stretching is good for arthritics—first, because it keeps the muscles at optimum length for highest efficiency (the cat needs to stretch before a long jump); second, because it keeps the joints loose by preventing muscle tightness; and third, because it helps reduce the chance of developing deformities as a result of abnormal muscle pull in combination with joint destruction.

Exercises to move the limbs as far as possible are called "range-of-motion exercises" (ROM) by physical therapists. When therapists speak of "stretching," they mean the same movements carried out passively beyond the range normally achieved by active motion without the therapist's help. In this stretching, the therapist does the work, moving the limb or other part of the body through its former range and slightly beyond without help from the patient.

It is usually not recommended for the patient to carry out such passive exercises himself, since he may not be able to judge when he exceeds the desirable range, something therapists are trained to observe. I have adopted some techniques used by therapists and have translated them into active exercise for the patient. I prefer to call them "stretching" even though no passive stretching is involved.

## RANGE OF MOTION

You should be very clear about the meaning of the words "full range of motion." The purpose of *daily* exercises is to maintain our original, normal range of motion. With the arm, for instance, we raise the arm straight over the head, out to the side, and down and backward as far as possible. These daily exercises are a preventive measure. Once the range has been noticeably reduced, which we see by our reduced function and may have confirmed by a therapist, we have to do *therapeutic* exercises for that particular part of the body. The task becomes more difficult and time-consuming, but it pays off by helping to prevent deformity, maintain function, and lessen pain. The slightest decrease in range is the signal for you to start correc-

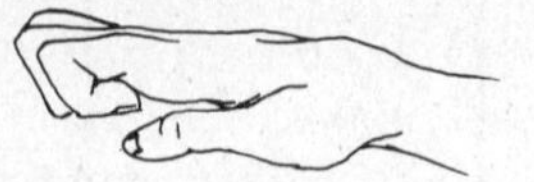

7. *The proper range for the intrinsic muscles is achieved in this position.*

tive exercises. The proper range for the intrinsic (small) muscles of the hand is achieved by the position shown in figure 7.

## ISOMETRICS AND ISOTONICS

We distinguish between *isometric exercises,* during which the joints are not moved, and *isotonic exercises,* during which the joints are moved. During an *active* exercise, muscles are exerted. In a *passive* exercise, muscles are relaxed and parts of the body are moved, for instance, with the help of a therapist or by the force of gravity. Nerve signals from and to the muscles can be stimulated and controlled in such a way as to permit the widest possible range of motion of the joints.

Most of our body activities require a combination of isometric and isotonic contractions. For instance, handling objects consists mostly of adjusting the grasp of the hand (isotonic), then holding the object (isometric).

## ISOMETRICS UPDATED

Isometric exercises were the subject of great public interest in the 1960s. All you had to do was to press your arms sideways against the frame of a door, your hands against a desk top, your legs against a chair, and so forth, for the brief "maximum" isometric contraction. This fad occurred after isometric training started to be analyzed scientifically in Germany in the middle fifties. The interest waned when athletes and trainers could not confirm that brief isometric exercises, consisting of only a few seconds of muscle contraction, could replace the much more time-consuming and strenuous training methods of the past.

In the meantime, scientific analysis has continued, and permits these efficient exercises to be utilized in a rational way. This is especially important in the management of arthritis, since isometric exercises are carried out with very little or no movement of any joint. A number of works published in the last decade (see Bibliography) have given us a better understanding of how isometric exercises work, and how they can be done both efficiently and conveniently to obtain optimum results. A full understanding permits us to design our own setup for exercise without blindly following instructions. I will describe these exercises in cookbook detail; with proper understanding you can translate these same exercises for one muscle group into efficient exercises for another.

## THE FORMULA FOR STRENGTHENING

I have said that I believe it is helpful to understand fully the physiological basis for exercises. Although you need not master the following explanation of muscle-strengthening, you may find it surprising and informative reading nonetheless.

The principle involved in muscle strengthening is to stimulate the growth of the muscle fibers through a muscle contraction stronger than the one used in normal activities. One daily maximum contraction of 1 second permits the muscle to gain its maximum possible strength within six weeks. One daily maximum contraction of 6 seconds shortens the time to about five weeks; several daily maximum contractions, for a total of 30 seconds, achieves maximum strengthening in four weeks; and a once-daily contraction at two-thirds maximum strength, lasting 1 second, requires eight and a half weeks to arrive at maximum strength. These results were reported for normal people starting with 80 percent of their strength potential. This means they added 20 percent strength and reached their limit in from four weeks to eight and a half weeks, depending on the frequency, length, and power of the daily contractions.

The question arises here, *what is a maximum contraction?* According to Erich A. Müller, a maximum muscular effort is one that cannot be maintained for more than about 12 seconds. It corresponds to about three times the strength at which a muscle is normally used. Double the normal strength produces a fair degree of isometric strengthening, even though it is not quite as strengthening as maximum effort. A one-time daily effort of 2–3 seconds, at maximum effort, is supposed to produce the biggest possible result in strengthening. Exercising at twice the normal effort (equivalent to two-thirds of the maximum effort) requires 6 seconds of effort, which can be distributed over several periods—for instance, two times at 3 seconds (count of six) each.

In the paper " 'Hand Gym' for Patients with Arthritic Hand Disabilities: Preliminary Report, 1978, an increase of about 20 percent was reported for the average strength of finger muscles after sixteen weeks. The exercises were done twice daily for 2–3 seconds (or a count of six) by pressing fingers as strongly as possible against the sides or bars of the Hand Gym. These being unsupervised exercises, I estimate that patients probably exercised to one-half or one-third of their maximum strength. It can be assumed that the normal strength exerted in daily activities corresponds to approximately one-sixth of the maximum force (this is the force that can be maintained for not more than 6 seconds). Isometric strengthening can be achieved, therefore, by exerting only twice the normal strength for 2–3 seconds daily. This is the clinical recommendation of Dr. Theodor Hettinger, who, together with Dr. Müller, has laid the groundwork for our understanding of the rationale of isometric exercise, and it has shown itself to be quite efficient in finger exercises.

Theoretically, the same regimen of twice-daily exercises of 2–3 seconds' duration, contracting as strongly as possible (i.e., two to three times the normally used strength, being equivalent to one-third to one-half maximum strength), should be sufficient to exercise all other skeletal muscles. If the muscles are very weak due to prolonged nonuse, as after bed rest, their strength increase will be fairly rapid at first, slowing down as you come closer to reaching the potential limit.

When daily training is stopped, the gain will be lost again in about the same period of time that was required to gain it—unless exercises are continued at least once a week or once every two weeks. Even at this rate, the muscle strength will eventually settle at the limit dictated by the condition of our joints. The study with the Hand Gym showed that eighteen patients with rheumatoid arthritis gained about 20 percent in strength in four months, as well as a satisfactory increase in function; the latter was due also to an increase in flexibility—that is, in the ranges of the small finger joints.

After four years, the eighteen patients with rheumatoid arthritis, and five with osteoarthritis who also went through the four months' training period, reported that they were satisfied with their strength and flexibility and hand function. Objective tests showed that the osteoarthritic patients had maintained half of the gain in strength after four months' training period (double the flexibility range gain which they had achieved in the four months). The rheumatoid patients fell back to their original strength (maintained half their gain in range of flexibility). All the patients reported exercising with the Hand Gym during the four-year period—some once or twice a week, some once every two weeks, some daily when they felt they needed it; the average was once weekly.

I learned from this that exercises done once or twice weekly on a regular basis are of benefit to maintain strength. This happens to conform to the results of studies reported by Müller. He found that a one-time weekly isometric workout in normal persons helps to maintain the strength required in daily work, thereby preventing fatigue. Thus, if we give our muscles a workout on the weekend, it gets us well through the week with our work. In addition, a yearly vacation of several weeks' duration, during which our muscles get a good workout, tones us up for the year ahead.

Apparently, the longer the training period is, the longer the gain in muscle strength remains with us. It seems therefore unnecessary to exercise several times daily to a total of 30 seconds for each muscle. As a matter of fact, the 6-second exercise may be somewhat taxing if carried out for each finger muscle. This would extend the five-minute daily workout with the Hand Gym to ten minutes. Considering that you may also want to strengthen other muscles of your arms, trunk, hips, legs, and feet, the total time expended for exercises would become taxing.

If one is told to exercise each finger muscle for 6 seconds (count of twelve), there may be a tendency not to try to reach a maximum contraction immediately, in order to hold through the full 6 seconds. This is just what we want to avoid. We want to get the best advantage from isometric exercises by keeping them brief. Two to three seconds (count of six) has been shown to be quite acceptable with finger muscles. In this period of time, one can also gain confidence that one exercised each muscle to a so-called maximum (in reality, probably only half the maximum).

# 5
# What to Do About Pain and Stiffness

When we are young, we tend to dismiss pain, to suppress it mentally, or to "tough it out." If it doesn't go away, we might take aspirin. After strenuous sports, we can usually heal our aches with a hot shower and a rubdown. We know that our body will repair itself in time. If I suffered a sprained ankle when jumping or mountain climbing, I knew that a properly applied bandage would ease the pain and all would be well again in a few days.

When I contracted arthritis, however, I learned that pain could be excruciating, unlike anything I had known before—perhaps with the exception of a toothache. But an extremely painful joint cannot be treated like a tooth; it doesn't help to tough it out and take a couple of aspirin tablets.

It took me quite a few years after the onset of the disease to radically change my attitude toward pain. I started to understand that the self-repairing ability of the muscles, tendons, ligaments, and other structures around the joints is diminished in arthritis. I have learned to observe—even to anticipate—every little twinge of pain occurring near the joints, and to take the right physical measures to heal the hurt and to prevent it from becoming worse. In my youth I would have looked on such behavior as hypochondria. But now that I have rheumatoid arthritis I respect the first twinges of pain. I know that if the cause is not removed the twinges often develop into much more persistent pains.

I believe (based on my own experience) that most arthritic pain develops slowly enough to be nipped in the bud before it develops into the kind of excruciating pain that requires instant use of very powerful medications. The inability to deal preventively, or therapeutically, with pain after it has settled in produces disabilities and depressions which may prevent us from taking effective measures to get back on our feet.

## PROS AND CONS OF PAINKILLERS

When the pain of arthritis is overwhelming, all one wants to do is grab for a painkiller. If you are using drugs in the management of pain, you will, of course, be doing so under the guidance of your physician. I do feel it can be helpful, though, to review certain of the other consequences—aside from freedom from pain—that go with the use of drugs. Often it comes as a surprise to arthritics that painkillers and other medications actually add to the stress in their lives and interfere with general healthy living.

The problem with painkillers is twofold, First, there is the appearance of harmful side effects—the slow stomach bleeding caused by aspirin ingestion, the narcotic effects of codeine, and the lasting and deleterious side effects of cortisone, which have now made it rare as a continuous treatment. Your physician will weigh these considerations carefully before prescribing medication, especially cortisone, which, when overused, can cause problems worse than the disease itself.

Furthermore, when an anti-inflammatory agent like cortisone is injected into a joint, it can produce a temporary pain-free euphoria during which we can seriously damage a joint. I once had a cortisone injection in my painful arthritic shoulder, after which I proceeded to saw a thick branch off a tree. The next day, the pain redoubled. It certainly *felt* as if I had damaged the joint.

Sleeping pills present yet a different problem, in that the effect of any one pill tends to be nullified after prolonged use, and you may find that you have come to depend on pills in order to be able to sleep. I agree that a good night's rest is essential for everyone, and especially for the arthritic, but I believe that purely physical means can go a long way toward inducing sound sleep. I discuss this at length in the next chapter. Try the tense-relax technique: tense each muscle of the body consecutively for 2 seconds, relax, tense the next muscle, relax, and so on.

## COMBATING CHRONIC PAIN

In some cases of pain and disability, surgical intervention is required to reconstruct or replace misshapen or misaligned joints. Usually, pain disappears after such procedures, but sometimes it lingers on. Cases in which all rational treatment has been exhausted and pain still persists can be called chronic pain cases. There have been many chronic pain clinics established throughout the country to deal with these problems. Many of the modalities used in such clinics are available also from the rehabilitation departments of major hospitals; some, however, are very new and are not yet available everywhere. These include such treatments as acupuncture and transcutaneous nerve stimulation (TNS); the latter is an electronic method of pain control which a patient can be taught to use at home. Other modalities include hypnosis and guided imagery, both of which are proving valuable in opposing pain through mind control.

In guided imagery the patient is taught to guide his imagination in pleasurable directions so that pain is displaced as the focus of attention. This brings to mind the case of Norman Cousins, former editor of the *Saturday Review*, who fought his otherwise intractable arthritis by setting up a deliberate program of viewing funny movies that would make him laugh for extended periods of time. The strategy succeeded, for reasons no one quite understands. I wonder if Mr. Cousins might have obtained some cleansing effect as the diaphragmatic and other muscular action associated with strong laughter stimulated his lymphatic system.

## GETTING AT THE CAUSE OF PAIN

I have used a great many of the available modalities in fighting my arthritis, including painkillers. During a bursitis attack that preceded the arthritis, I found that codeine allowed me to sleep.

During my first strong flare-up of rheumatoid arthritis, I got relief from Butazolidin. At later stages I had cortisone injections into my finger joints and the shoulder.

Learn, if you can, to anticipate painful episodes and to use physical means such as immobilization, heat, and exercise to deflect development of the pain. When I first read the principle that physical therapy ideally should be able to prevent a painful state, I did not understand it, nor did I believe it. Now, after seventeen years of living with arthritis, I have a fuller grasp of the meaning of this principle. I am trying to communicate in this book the various exercises you can use to combat pain along with other modalities. I am gratefull for all strong painkillers with which I was treated, and I acknowledge their value in decreasing pain and making it possible to increase range through exercise. But the less of them you use, and the more the pain is eliminated through physical means, the more comfortable you will be.

What I offer my readers is the optimism I have that something can be done to help alleviate and remove the cause of each arthritic hurt in any part of our body. Learning where the pain comes from helps us to decide how to deal with it. We will not always necessarily succeed with the first modality we try. But if one doesn't work, another one will.

## TO REDUCE INFLAMMATION

Before discussing other modalities of pain management, let me repeat that most of the pain in rheumatoid arthritis is due to inflammation. The inflammation in the joint is accompanied by a considerable thickening of the synovium, the membrane that encloses the joint space. At the same time, there is a tendency for fluid to be retained in and around the joint. The pressure of the liquid and of the synovium against adjacent ligaments and against the capsule which surrounds the joint produces pain as ligaments and/or the capsule is stretched and twisted. Inflammation also occurs along tendons which cross the joints. Tendons are covered by synovial sheaths which are also liable to become inflamed so that pain is felt at points along the tendon.

If the inflammation was not contained sufficiently by the drug regimen, as becomes evident from the pain, the following physical means are available to fight it: (1) rest, (2) heat, (3) gentle movements to dissipate stagnant liquid, and (4) exercises.

## REST

Rest can be provided for joints or tendons in several ways. The painful joint or painful part of the tendon is immobilized by a splint; if a splint is not available, an Ace bandage can be used. Immobilization is particularly useful overnight, to prevent the slight movements during sleep that tend to irritate the joint. (Think of a broken bone. It will never heal if you simply rest in the hope of not moving it. You have to set it in a cast in order for it to heal.) The fact that immobilization helps has been amply described in medical literature and I have experienced it very successfully. I have never read a satisfactory explanation for this effect. One factor contributing to inflammation may be the disturbance of the tiny lymph channels near the joints. Complete immobilization may help to restore efficient flow through these channels, and as liquid clears from the inflamed area, there is less pressure on pain-sensitive structures.

*Morning stiffness* is typical in arthritis. It is usually due to the accumulation of fluids in or near the joints during the night. The length of time it lasts after you arise from bed is a good measure for the degree of activity of the disease. It subsides after a while because you move about after you get up, and the movements of the body tend to cause the accumulated fluids to dissipate. A warm bath in the morning during which you move about—using soap, rinsing, and drying oneself—speeds up the disappearance of morning stiffness through the combination of heat and gentle motion. I feel the very important exercises to maintain and increase joint range should be done *after* the bath or after the morning stiffness has subsided in other ways, so that their main purpose—namely, moving your extremities through the largest range possible—will not be hindered.

*Gelling,* a phenomenon similar to stiffness, can occur after you have been sitting quietly without moving for a long time, especially in a draft. It can happen also if you have been clutching a telephone tightly during a lengthy conversation; you seem to have a hard time letting go of the receiver. If you notice these effects, make sure that you move frequently while you sit, especially your feet and ankles. Also, shift the telephone receiver from hand to hand several times during a long conversation. The so-called gelling is not specifically indicative of arthritis; people generally are liable to become stiff if they sit for extended periods of time, as during intercontinental air travel.

## WHY REST AND EXERCISE?

Here I will remind you of the chief reason why we exercise to obtain relief from pain. Through exercises we can keep a joint in proper alignment and so reduce the stress on ligaments. A joint is usually stabilized in part of its range by muscles and in another part by ligaments. If the joint is used in that part of the range which relies on muscle power, less stress is going to be placed on ligaments; therefore, there will be less twisting or stretching of these ligaments (which are already weakened by the disease) and less pain.

The reader is justified in asking here, "Why are rest and movement both used to combat pain?" The answer is that they work in different ways. For reasons not yet fully understood, there seems to be some recovery from the process of deterioration during complete rest. When there is gentle movement, either active or passive, the flow of liquid through the larger lymph channels away from the joints is encouraged, thereby lessening pressure and promoting the removal of wastes. A muscle which contains metabolic products like lactic acid, which have not been cleared away, feels very painful. In the athlete, such a condition can result after a peak performance like the hundred-yard dash. By slow deliberate muscle action, these products are "pumped" out of the muscle, and that is why the athlete will run slowly in place for a time following an event. In the arthritic such a condition mostly arises when muscles go into spasm, working extra hard to protect a painful area. For instance, to prevent a vertebra from pinching a nerve, the muscle may contract to pull the vertebra to one side. In order for this muscle to be relieved of the metabolic product of this effort, it has to be exercised. But exercise may not be easy so long as the muscle is not relaxed. Relaxation can be achieved through heat (also through cold), massage, and immobilization of the concerned vertebra (for instance, by wearing a cervical collar).

Indirectly, pain can be produced when nerves are pinched or compressed due to the irregular pull of muscles and distortion of the supporting bones nearby. Such pain—for instance, sciatica pain in the lower back reaching down into the legs—can be very strong and disabling. Surrounding muscles have to be relaxed and exercised to reduce abnormal pulls.

All conditions of pain should be reported to your physician, so that you can decide together what modality to choose to combat it. Your physician also must make the extremely important determination of whether your pain is really caused by arthritis, or whether it comes from a pinched nerve or some completely different and unrelated condition. Sometimes these conditions are very difficult to tell apart.

## WHAT HEAT CAN DO

My rheumatologist told me at an early stage of my arthritis, "Heat is your best friend." An exact explanation of why heat works so well to reduce pain in arthritis is not yet conclusively established. One of the theories suggests that the pain-nerve endings send fewer pain signals to the brain when they are heated or cooled. This is why both heat and cold are usable modalities to reduce arthritis pain. However, both heat and cold, as they are administered for arthritis, also result in increased circulation, and this may have a salutary effect in clearing fluids from painful areas.

Heat applications are either wet or dry. In the first type, water in some form—perhaps a whirlpool bath or a steaming hot compress—is the conductor of the heat. Dry heat radiates from some nonhumid source, such as a heat lamp. Let us consider first the various applications of wet heat.

## FOMENTATIONS

Outside the bathroom I have used heat applications in the form of fomentations. For this you make a compress by dipping a folded towel in very hot water, then wringing it out and applying it over the joint. Cover it with a plastic sheet for insulation, and renew compress about every five minutes. So that the skin does not cool off between applications, it is useful to work with two compresses, applying one immediately after the other one has cooled off.

## ELECTRIC HOT PADS

A humid electric hot pad produces an effect somewhat similar to that of the hot compress. The pad I am using, called the Thermophore, available in surgical supply stores (price, about $50) is dry to start with, but sheds some humidity between the long, soft fibers of its cover while in use (the humidity, as I understand it, is extracted from the air). The pad gives out heat only while the pushbutton switch is kept depressed, and produces much stronger heat than one gets with the usual type of electric heating pads.

Many automatic electric heating pads are equipped with a flat sponge which can be dipped into water for a wet application. They produce a moister but less warm application than the Thermophore. Electric hot pads do not conform as well as compresses to round joints such as the knee, shoulder, or elbow. They work better on flat areas, such as the back and hips. Remember that in case of trouble with the lower back, *mild* heat is usually recommended.

## FOR PAINFUL HANDS

A treatment helpful for painful hands is to dip them into hot water for twenty minutes or so. I use a plastic bowl into which I run a slow but constant stream of water, as hot as I can stand it. I put about half a cup of epsom salts into the bowl, which contributes to heat conduction and helps protect the skin.

A small, hot whirlpool bath, fig. 7a permits a higher water temperature to be used for higher efficiency. The massaging action of the swirling water helps deflate swelling.

To prolong the feeling of comfort after a heat application, it helps to apply a rubbing ointment or liniment containing salicylic acid, menthol, or camphor.

The *paraffin treatment* for hands is usually administered in hospitals or clinics, since the heating of the paraffin has to be carefully supervised; it cannot be overheated or the patient may suffer burns. In this treatment, the hands are dipped completely into the hot paraffin bath. When the hands are withdrawn and cooled in the air, the thin layer of paraffin sets and hardens. The hands are dipped again briefly several times until a number of wax layers have built up, covering the hands like tight gloves. The hands with the paraffin "gloves" are then wrapped in a towel and rested for twenty minutes, after which the wax is removed. After such an application, my hands felt pleasantly warm and pain-free, but fairly stiff. I find a soak in hot water preferable, as it leaves my hands flexible and I am able to move my fingers during the treatment.

## DRY HEAT

Dry heat is another way of treating the pain of arthritis. In general I find heat lamps less efficient than wet applications. They produce localized hot areas on the skin which are susceptible to cool drafts, even in rooms at normal temperature. Dry heat from the sun, when taken in a dry climate, is extremely pleasant and makes the whole body feel good. In a humid climate sunbathing can be disagreeable, since the normal evaporation from the skin cannot take place due to the humidity; this alone results in discomfort. In addition, a draft or slight wind can produce cooling of localized perspired areas, and muscle spasms and further pain may result.

*Diathermy* and *ultrasound* are two modalities which also can be considered dry heat. They employ electromagnetic waves which are aimed inside the body. I had diathermy treatment prior to cortisone injections into the finger joints. The fifteen-minute treatment made my fingers feel warm and comfortable only while the application lasted. A close relative reports successful treatment with ultrasound for a bruise that did not go away after treatment with external hotpacks and local massage. Such modalities, now commonly used by dancers and athletes, are only available under close supervision of a physician.

## COLD APPLICATIONS

In recent years cold applications have become popular in the treatment of arthritic pain. Most arthritics shy away from anything cold, thinking it makes arthritis worse. However, the numbing effect of cold compresses reduces pain. The pain receptors in the skin becomes less sensitive with lower temperature; at first, there is reduced circulation in the area. Although this does not help to "heal" anything, the lower pain permits better movements of the joints. This is important. Cold can be applied by rubbing an ice cube over the area to be cooled or by applying an ice bag (available from drugstores, or you can make one by filling a plastic bag with crushed ice). Time of application: until numb, usually less than 20 minutes.

## PREPARING YOURSELF TO FIGHT PAIN

At first inkling that you may develop a persistent pain, "throw heat" at it immediately, or use any other modality recommended to fight it. The earlier you catch and eliminate pain, the more time you save in the long run. Hot packs, hot-water soaks, and whirlpool baths usually take twenty minutes to half an hour, and while you may resent the time involved, these measures have to be taken for therapeutic reasons, if you want to control a pain before it "settles in." "Working off" a pain that has settled in may take many months, as I experienced with my neck, jaw, back, and shoulders.

Hand-rest splints should always be kept available to be used immediately, when necessary, to immobilize a joint. Failing to do this could mean pain persisting throughout the next day indicating additional irritational damage, which will then take longer to remedy.

# PART II

## THE CHAPTERS

# 6
# Hand Exercises and Splints

Every joint in the body serves an important purpose in its own way, yet the hands, with their complex interplay of joints, seem particularly important to us. We use our hands all the time, which means that if we don't have the use of hands we are handicapped all the time.

In arthritis, the finger joints are attacked early, often before the disease is even diagnosed. In rheumatoid arthritis, the inflamed knuckles are vulnerable to destruction when fingers are used in their accustomed way; eventually the finger segments become twisted in odd directions and the fingers are unable to function for grasping. The muscles spanning the painful joints tend to waste, and as their supportive function lessens, deformities set in.

Medication helps to reduce inflammation and pain. However, a regimen of rest and exercises to strengthen the muscles can help delay the destruction of the knuckles by keeping the knuckles stabilized and minimizing abnormal pull. Fingers supported by strong muscles will not be immediately displaced when we lean against or carry an object with them.

The motions of the hands and wrists include flexion and extension, abduction and adduction, and internal and external rotation. Considering the very large number of finger joints, we might suppose that innumerable exercises would be needed to fully exercise them. This may well be the reason why comprehensive finger exercises were unavailable for so long. There were only a few standard exercises: making a fist, spreading the fingers apart; touching the tip of the thumb to the tips of the individual fingers; and placing the hand on a flat surface and lifting individual fingers. An exercise that arthritics should avoid is squeezing a rubber ball. It is destructive of the finger joints, and I personally find it inefficient, since pain in the knuckles prevents one from squeezing the rubber ball hard enough to produce strengthening effect. The only other exercises for hand and fingers I know of are the so-called etudes for the piano (or just plain piano-playing) and the various hand and finger positions used by dancers and Yoga practitioners, which are intended mainly to achieve flexibility.

## WHY AND HOW I DEVELOPED THE HAND GYM

In my case, my fingers became weak and clumsy one or two years before inflammation actually appeared. I lost the ability to use the precision tools that were necessary to my work. Turning a key in a lock became more difficult, and opening a food jar produced pain in the big knuckles. When inflammation of the knuckles began, I simply stopped using the painful fingers. As the inflammation subsided in these fingers and moved on to the other fingers, the whole hand gradually became very weak. During periods of remission for individual fingers, the muscles of these fingers never quite regained their strength since there was no way to train them individually, and the pain in the inflamed fingers made it very hard to do squeezing exercises for the whole hand. After about two years of the disease, my fingers seemed to stiffen at wrong angles, so that, besides lacking strength, they were now *unable* to grip things properly. I could no longer use a knife and fork, nor could I button my shirt or tie my shoelaces. My rheumatologist sent me to a hand surgeon who outlined to me the possibility of fusing some of the joints; the suggested procedure would also have "released" the overly strong contracture of some of the muscles to permit a better grip—though not necessarily more strength. (Nowadays finger joints can be replaced with Silastic rubber implants, which produce a good-looking hand but only limited improvement in strength, if any.) I therefore studied the possibility of deliberate exercises to loosen some of my tight muscles, which seemed preferable to the so-called surgical release, by which some of the muscle mass or the associated tendinous structure would be removed and the muscles rendered less effective. I wanted to preserve the muscles to the greatest extent possible. I also realized that after an operation, strengthening would have to be done through deliberate exercise anyway. I worked out my own exercise system, designing an apparatus which my wife, Elsa, put together according to my instructions out of cardboard, bolts, rubber bands, and foam rubber. I called it the Hand Gym (figure 8). By placing my fingers in the straight slots, I counteracted their tendency to deviate in the direction of the little finger (ulnar deviation). I could press my fingers against the walls of the slots on both sides to increase strength. The bolts that pass through the walls at right angles provide support for the fingers to counteract the direction of deformity; that is, if the first segment beyond the large knuckles developed a tendency flexion, the bolt would support this segment in the extended position. Where the middle segment seemed to want to hyperextend or point upward (swan-neck deviation), I exercised the finger by trying to curl it around a foam-rubber roll.

Exercises of a few minutes' duration, several times a day, resulted in my regaining sufficient strength and flexibility to be able once again to feed and dress myself. I have maintained this ability now for fourteen years even though my hands are reduced in strength. Apparently, I was able to retard the process

**8.** *The Hand Gym provides slots to permit fingers to be pressed sideways against its walls.*

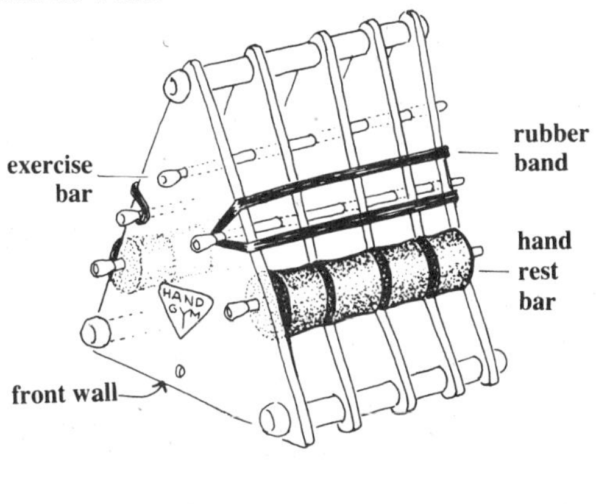

of deformation and retain sufficient strength, although it is limited by the destruction the joints have suffered. We arthritics have to "live within the limitations" dictated by our joints. However, maintaining flexibility goes far in substituting for strength.

## THE CLINICAL STUDIES

My rheumatologist was very pleased with the results I had obtained with the Hand Gym and asked me to explain the system to the doctors at the Institute of Rehabilitation Medicine at New York University Medical Center in New York City. The occupational therapy department and the clinical director of the Institute, Dr. Edward Lowman, were quite excited about the possibilities of this exercise system. They undertook a two-year clinical study during which a booklet with detailed descriptions of the exercises was compiled by Doris Bens, an occupational therapist at the institute. The Hand Gym was then modified to fit the various sizes of hands, and one hundred were produced. At the institute it was also found that the exercises benefited people with weakness or partial paralysis from conditions other than arthritis, including strokes, fractures, burns, and hand surgery. A manufacturer was found and today the Hand Gym is distributed through surgical and medical supply houses throughout the United States and in many countries around the world (catalogue number F70900, Maddak Inc., and Arthritis Aids Div. (see Dir. of Aids). The instructions are available in ten languages.

The exercises in this chapter are designed to be done with the Hand Gym. If you are in treatment, ask your doctor or therapist to supervise your first exercise session. In a few instances, the principles behind certain exercises can be adapted for exercising without the Hand Gym. I am offering this system to my readers here because, as I have said, it is the only fully balanced regimen of hand exercises that I know of.

While the instructions were being compiled at the institute, I did some studies of the electrical impulses of finger muscles during their contraction to see in what directions isometric contractions (without joint motion) would be most efficient for strengthening. I also dissected hands together with my rheumatologist, Dr. Otto Steinbrocker, at New York University Medical School to get more insight into the function of finger muscles. I did extensive bibliographical research on finger deformities and exercises in arthritis and presented a summary of my design and analysis to Dr. Adrian Flatt, a renowned hand surgeon who specializes in arthritis cases. In his critique, he supported the concept and advised me to have a clinical study done and to publish the results. Dr. Steinbrocker referred me for this purpose to St. Vincent's Hospital in New York City, where Dr. Samuel Sverdlik, head of the rehabilitation department, supervised a clinical study of twenty-three carefully screened arthritis patients—eighteen with rheumatoid arthritis and five with osteoarthritis. Six to eight months passed between the time the patients applied for the study and the time the study was started. This represented a control period during which their hand disabilities continued and no Hand Gym exercises were done. After this, the patients embarked on a four-month program of twice-daily exercising with the Hand Gym. At the beginning and at monthly intervals, the chief occupational therapist at St. Vincent's, Anita Simmons, took strength and flexiblity measurements and checked the patients' ability to do certain functional jobs—turning a key in a lock, opening a jar, picking up small objects, and so forth. The supervising physician, Dr. Judith Schauffler, saw the patients on the same days and evaluated their progress. At the end of the study, the majority of the rheumatoid arthritis patients and all of the osteoarthritis patients exhibited increased flexibility and strength as well as improvement in their function. Several could close their fists completely, which they had not been able to do before, and thus they were able once again to hold eating utensils of regular design rather than the type with built-up handles used by many arthritics.

As long as we can manage without such compensating devices as built-up handles, I believe we are much better off to do so, since they make life very much more complicated.

I am grateful for the roughly fourteen years of reasonably normal use of my hands that I have had since developing the Hand Gym and I look forward to continued functioning. I am also convinced that if I had started this exercise system much earlier during my arthritis, my hands would have been better protected and would be less deformed than they are today. I believe that such exercises help to educate the hand to function in a protective position which minimizes the stress on joints. If this protective position is carried over from exercise sessions into daily life, joints are less liable to suffer destruction.

## THE GOAL IS JOINT PROTECTION

The philosophy of *joint protection* is really the mainstay of physical and occupational therapy for the arthritic hand. The most important elements of joint protection are:

1. Educating the hand to function in a position that places minimal stress on the joints.
2. Exercising to keep fingers flexible and strong in order to maintain the favorable position.
3. Splinting of the hand to reduce inflammation and, if need be, to prevent positions that produce deformity.

Please note, however, that hand exercises are not intended to strengthen the hand to the point where it becomes capable of destroying its own joints in use. The clinical study showed that in rheumatoid arthritics, strengthening occurs to the highest degree in those fingers or in those particular muscles that have lost most of their strength. Thus a proper balance is reestablished.

As clinical studies have shown, strengthening exercises have to be done daily only for a period of a few months; after that, only when the need for them is felt but at least once weekly. Range-of-motion exercises to maintain or increase flexibility should be done daily, however.

## ANATOMY OF THE HAND

Before proceeding to describe the exercises, it will be helpful to study the following drawings of the hand to familiarize ourselves with the anatomical names of the various bones and

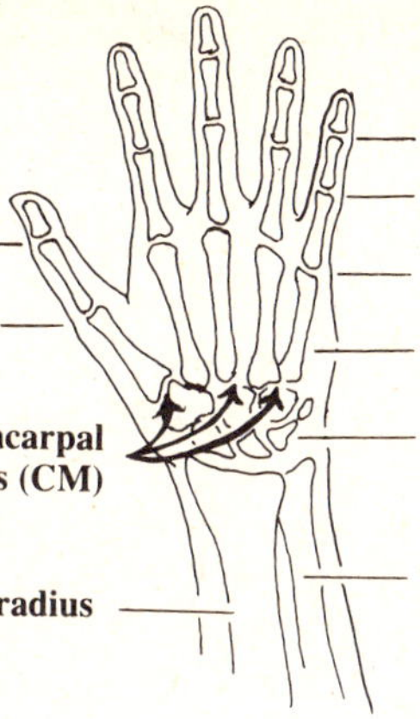


**9.** *Anatomical names for joints and bones of the hands.*

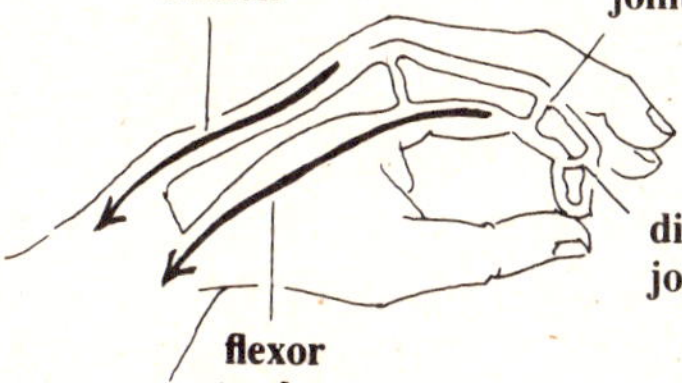


**9a.** *Function of hand joints when grasping an object between the tip of the finger and the thumb.*

joints (figures 9 and 9a). Occupational therapists who deal with arthritics try to teach these terms to their patients to facilitate communication about bones, joints, deformities, protective positions, exercise positions, and so forth. (Figure 5, page 44, shows direction of pull of the various hand muscles.)

## TESTING THE HAND AND WRIST RANGES

First, let us test your fingers and hands for flexibility. These are the types of tests my rheumatologist asks me to perform during my biannual checkups. If any of the ranges are limited, it is important to try to regain them by daily exercise.

- Spread the fingers of both hands far apart (figure 10). The fingers have to be straight. If you are at the point in your arthritis where you cannot straighten your fingers, use a support such as the edge of a table or the Hand Gym.
- Touch the tip of the thumb to the base of the little finger (figure 11). If you cannot quite do this, rotate and circle the thumb a few times to warm it, then try again.
- Curl the fingers with the tips of the fingers touching the base of the fingers with the MCP (big knuckle) straight (figure 12) so that the palm is flat and does not show wrinkles. If you cannot manage this, practice the exercise with the Hand Gym (see figures 36 and 37, page 100). Finger-curling without and with resistance will help. This is a very important test. If you cannot do it properly, it means that the very disabling *swan-neck* deformity (see figure 24, page 88) could be in the process of forming.

Until recently, physicians merely wanted you to show that you could make a fist (figure 13), but this is not a sufficient test of your flexibility. Also, please do not consider the making of a fist an adequate exercise; it does not place certain very important small muscles under stretch.

When the MCP joint is flexed, a large amount of muscle power is concentrated to pull the proximal phalanx into flexion, and this could produce subluxation (partial dislocation) of the joint (see figure 26, page 88) if the joint is not properly stabilized by its collateral ligaments. In rheumatoid arthritis these ligaments are subject to stretch, and subluxation of the MCP joint results. That is why we want to "train the hand" in using a protective position (figure 14) for grasping objects in daily life as well as during exercises. In this position, the MCP joint is kept extended and the PIP and DIP joints are flexed. It is bad to bend the MCP joint during the grasp (figure 15).

If you cannot make a fist, don't force it. It could do harm by placing undue stress on the ligaments of the MCP joints. Instead, exercise as shown in figure 37 (see page 100) to keep fingers flexible.

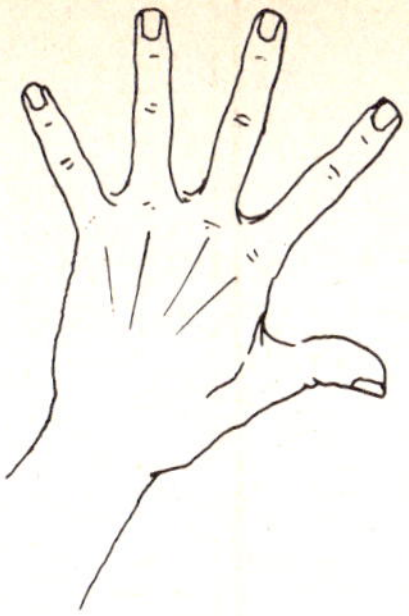

**10.** *Spread fingers as far apart as possible.*

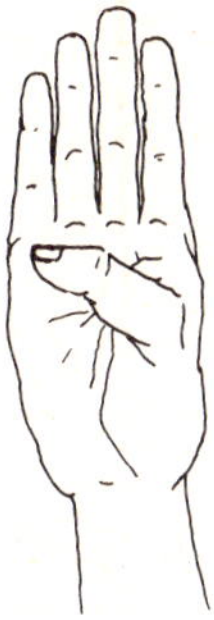

**11.** *Touch tip of thumb to base of little finger.*

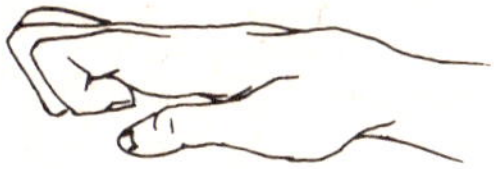

**12.** *Curl fingers so that tips touch the base of the fingers. Keep the large knuckles straight.*

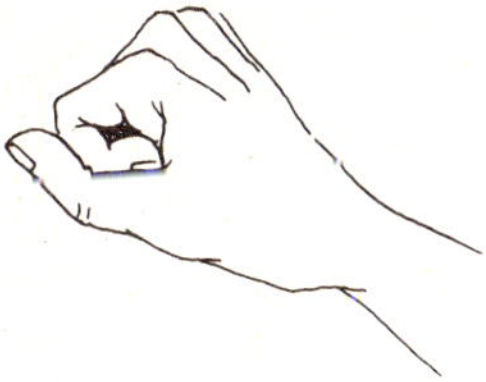

**13.** *Making a fist.*

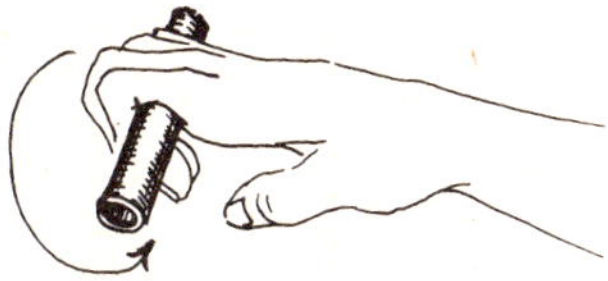

**14.** *Correct protective position for grasping objects. Extend MCP and PIP; flex DIP.*

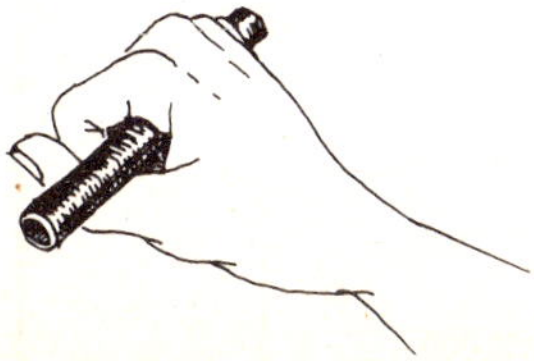

**15.** *Incorrect position for grasping. The MCP joint should not be bent.*

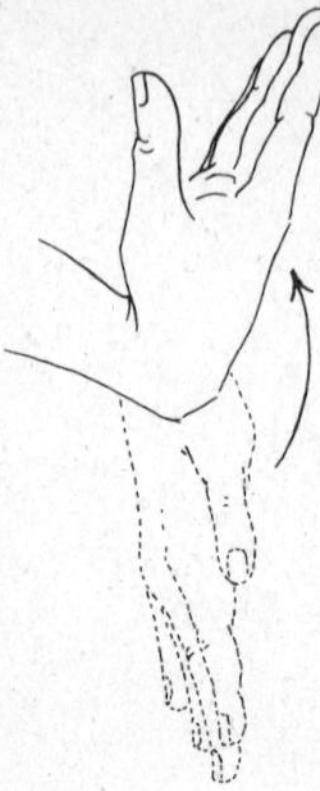

**16.** *Extend both wrists, upward.*

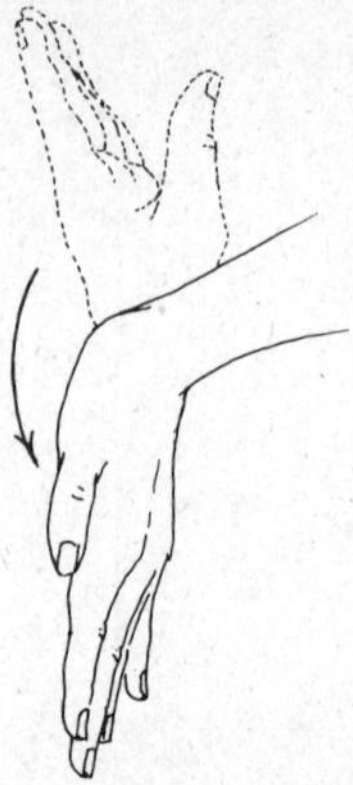

**17.** *Flex both wrists, downward.*

The ranges of motion of the wrists usually are evaluated at the same time as the fingers. A full range of wrist motion is important for two reasons. First, the muscles whose tendons span the wrists are placed under slight stretch as the wrist is articulated. The finger flexors are stretched when the wrist is extended (figure 16) and the finger extensors when the wrist is flexed (figure 17). This slight stretch makes the muscle more efficient. Similar considerations hold true for the other motions of the wrists.

Second, the various motions of the wrists are necessary in everyday life. They come into play when we are shaving, brushing our teeth, stirring a pot, bathing, putting on clothes. Restricted motion of the wrist is very hampering.

Test the wrist ranges in the following way:

- Abduct both wrists by turning them out; adduct both wrists by turning them inward (figure 18). Extend both wrists all the way by turning them up (figure 16) and

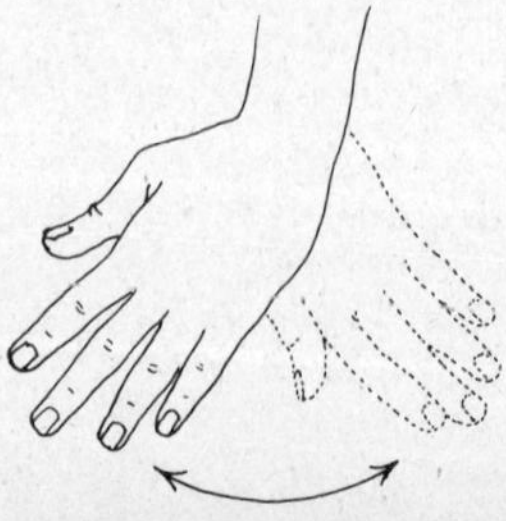

**18.** *Turn both hands out (abduct) and in (adduct).*

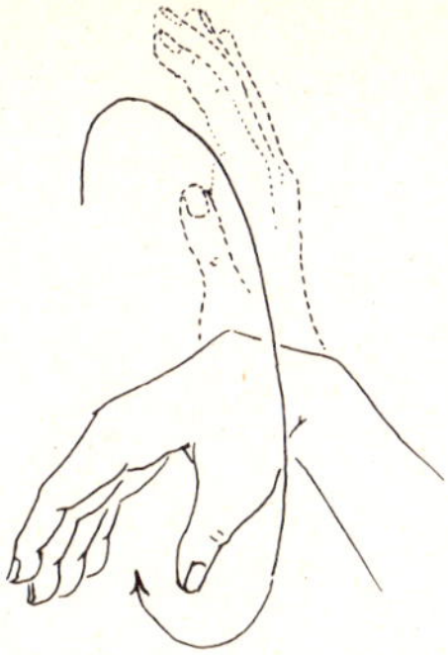

**19.** *Rotate both wrists in the largest circle possible. Circle in both directions.*

flex both wrists out by turning them all the way down (figure 17).

The drawings show the limits of the ranges that should be obtained. If you exercise and don't reach these limits, move slowly, tighten your wrist muscles for about two seconds, relax, and turn further.

- Rotate the wrists (figure 19). During evaluation of this exercise, note whether you develop any pain in doing this with the largest circle possible. If so, stop just before the point of pain, contract the muscles, relax, and circle once or twice again.
- *Pronate* the hands by rotating the forearms and wrists so that the palms of the hands are down. Then *supinate* the hands so that the palms of the hands are up (figure 20).

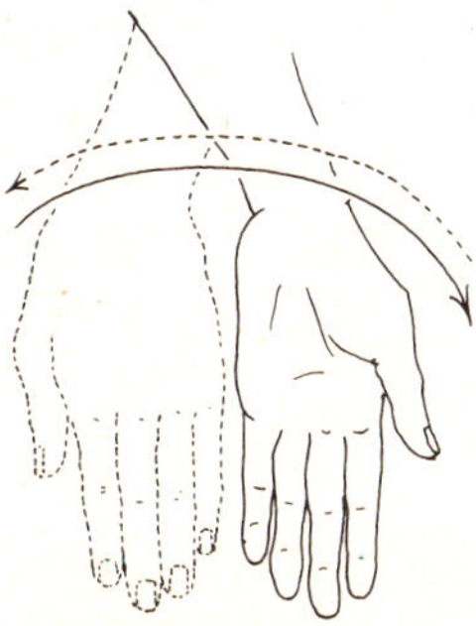

**20.** *Pronate and supinate the hands, by turning hands and forearm together, in and out.*

## HAND DEFORMITIES

If the following discussion of hand deformities seems too complex for you to go into at this point, you can skip it and proceed with the description of Hand Gym Exercises. Knowledge of the kinesiology, or function, of the hand and of deformities is not necessary in order to carry out exercise properly, but some readers may be interested in the subject.

Everybody, however, should be fully aware of the importance of the protective position of the hand (figure 21), which is used in the Hand Gym exercises, and then carried over into daily life.

In the normal use of the hand—that is, the way the hand is used by a normal person without disabilities—the phalanges are usually first moved into a position so that they clear the object to be grasped. This means the hand is opened sufficiently to accommodate the object. Next, the fingers are bent to conform to the surface of the object to be grasped. Finally, the object is grasped and held. The motions of the fingers and individual phalanges involved are flexion, extension, abduction, adduction, and rotation.

The fingers are moved by so-called *extrinsic* and *intrinsic* hand muscles. The powerful extrinsics are located in the forearm and send their tendons through your wrist to attach to the various phalanges. When you hold your hand over your knee, and press into the knee with your fingertips or with the middle phalanges, you can feel by touching the lower part of your forearm how the flexor muscles bulge as you exert pressure on your knee. When you straighten your hand out against the underside of a table you can feel the extrinsic extensor muscles in the back of your forearm; these are the antagonists to the much stronger flexors.

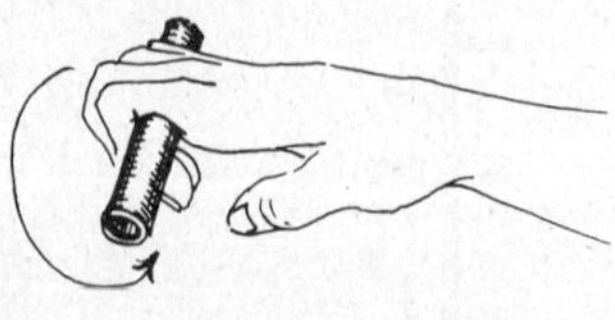

**21.** *Correct protective position for grasping objects. Extend MCP and PIP; flex DIP.*

The intrinsic mucles are located within the hand itself. Most of them are hard to detect as they are located right between the bones. They are called interossei (meaning "between bones"). Together with the extrinsic extensors, they help to abduct, adduct, and rotate the fingers. One of the interossei, a very important one called dorsal interosseus No. 1, can be observed between the roots of the index finger and the thumb. When you abduct the index finger strongly against resistance you can feel the belly of this muscle contracting if you touch it with a fingertip of the other hand.

## Ulnar Deviation

The interosseus No. 1 is a very important muscle. It keeps the index finger from slipping into the ulnar direction (that is, the direction away from the thumb and toward the ulna, the outer bone of the forearm) when pressure is placed on the side of the index finger, as in turning a key in a lock. This immediately gives us an idea where the very common *ulnar deviation* deformity comes from. (In figure 22, all fingers, not only the index finger, are deviating in the direction of the ulna.) A hand-rest splint helps to control it (figure 23).

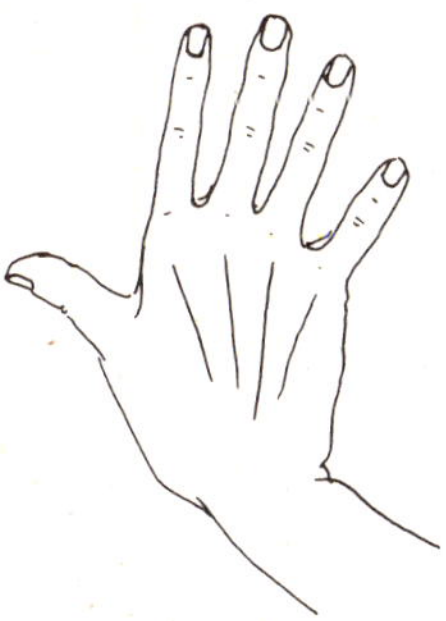

**22.** *Ulnar deviation. Fingers off to the side.*

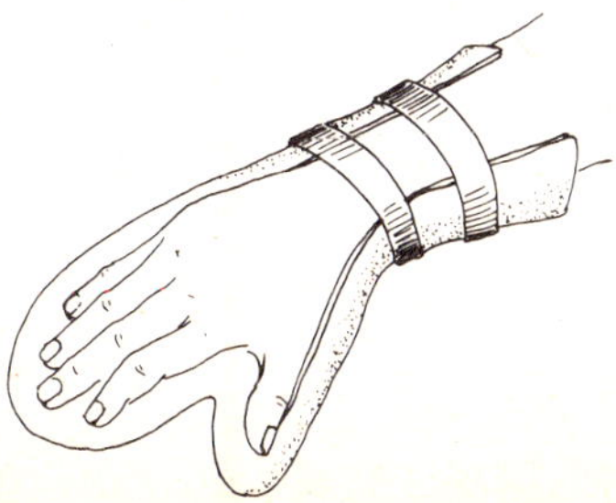

**23.** *Hand-rest splint. Wear it at night to reduce inflammation and to control ulnar deviation if present.*

As long as fingers remain flexible, this ulnar deviation does not present much of a handicap, except that you lose the ability to oppose the tips of the little finger and the thumb. It results in a slight decrease of dexterity of which many old people, even those without arthritis, complain. However, once you permit your fingers to become stiff in those positions of deformity, they are liable to become nonfunctional. The difficulty with this deformity and with subluxation (see page 88) is that if the condition goes untreated it will prevent you from flattening out your hand, making it difficult to open the hand sufficiently to grasp large objects. And once you lose the ability to grasp, your hand very quickly becomes weaker and stiffer just because you don't use it much. It is very important to keep the hands flexible so that these two types of deformities, namely ulnar deviation and the subluxation of the MCP joints, do not interfere with your function.

My hands, after seventeen years of arthritis, show both of these conditions in a very pronounced way; however, my fingers are very flexible, and although my hands are not as strong as they used to be, they can carry out practically all functions I require of them. I do make use of two devices that permit me to get better leverage and so reduce the strain on my finger joints. These are a key holder and a jar opener (see Dir. of Aids).

I am dismayed to read exercise instructions for arthritic hands that call for repeated turning of keys in locks and operation of jar openers as a means of strengthening your fingers. I can state from my own experience that as you lose the power to turn a key in a lock or to open a jar, you automatically want to repeat these motions again and again in order not to lose those functions. This same holds true, for instance, when making a complete fist. However, the results are miserable. The painful joints which produce the weakness in the first place become even more painful. Such exercises, it seems to me, don't take into account the causes of pain, particularly joint misalignment and muscle imbalance.

Deliberate isometric exercises for the individual muscle in positions in which the joints are supported and protected, as in the Hand Gym, produce the desired results. I noticed this myself after a few months' use of the Hand Gym; it was also observed with most patients in the Hand Gym study who had these functional complaints. It seems paradoxical that you should still use mechanical devices once the strength has been regained to the point where you can use a key or unscrew a jar; however, you want to place a minimum amount of stress on your joints in order to preserve them. The additional strength obtained in the exercises here is useful first to stretch tight intrinsic muscles through finger-curling, and second, to create muscle balance around the various finger joints so that any pressure in any direction on the fingers will be distributed uniformly, producing a minimum of stress on ligaments weakened through disease.

This principle can be graphically illustrated in connection with quadriceps muscle of the thigh. When I developed difficulty in climbing stairs, my therapist told me to strengthen the quadriceps muscles, which extend the knee. They had become very weak after several months of bed rest due to an illness not connected with arthritis. Before I consulted the therapist, I tried to force myself to climb stairs but was severely limited in this by pain in my knees. This was not necessarily arthritic pain; it was probably due to undue strain on ligaments that were called upon to stabilize the knee in the absence of sufficiently strong muscle power. After two weeks of concentrated quadriceps muscle exercises, climbing stairs became very easy and the knee pain was gone. Some of my readers, who may have already observed the need for quadriceps exercise, will be able to transfer the principle behind the knee exercises to finger exercises—namely, that strengthening muscles around joints stabilizes the joints, reduces joint pain by making it possible to use the joints more efficiently, and improves function.

## Swan-Neck Deformity

In the very disabling deformity called *swan neck,* the middle phalanx rides up instead of continuing in a straight line with the proximal phalanx. The distal phalanx is flexed but cannot grip

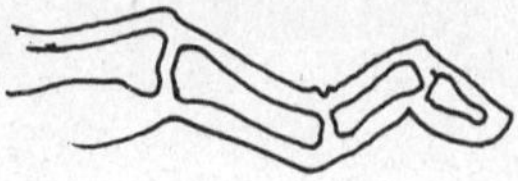

**24.** *Swan-neck deformity.*

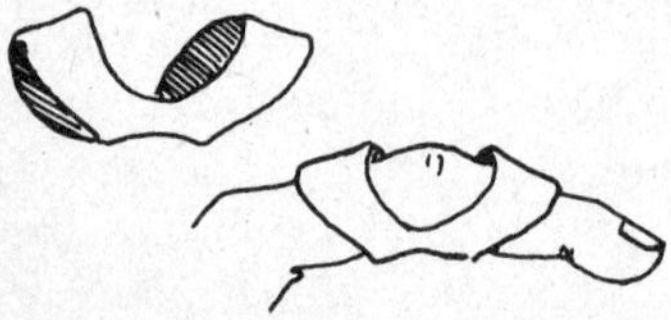

**25.** *Swan-neck ring. A splint to help finger bend properly.*

objects (figure 24). A splint to control the deformity is shown in figure 25. Among the factors contributing to this deformity is the abnormal pull (contracture) of intrinsic muscles, which prevents you from curling the fingers as indicated in figure 21 on page 84, with the MCP joints (big knuckles) straight. Eventually, the middle phalanx cannot be flexed at all, and if there is some damage to the structure around the PIP joint, the middle phalanx will ride up in an abnormal way. The distal phalanx will flex automatically due to abnormal tendon pull, but the unnatural position of the proximal phalanx makes it impossible to grasp anything with this flexed distal phalanx. The finger will eventually become stiff from disuse in this abnormal position.

*Subluxation* of the MCP joint (figure 26) is another contributing factor in the swan-neck deformity. This subluxation displaces the tendon of the intrinsic muscles in such a way as to produce an effect similar to muscle contracture (shortening). In subluxation the muscle is not shortened, but the tendon has to reach around the subluxed base of the proximal phalanx, so that there is not enough slack for the tendons to bend around the proximal phalanx. In my personal experience with my severely subluxed right hand, I was able to keep the proximal phalanx flexible enough through exercise of the type shown in figure 37

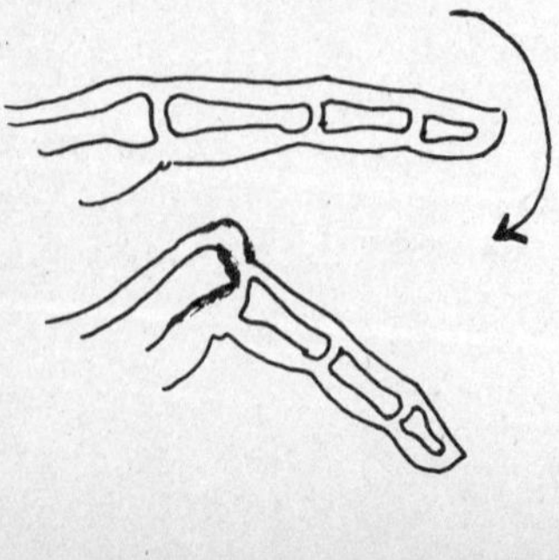

**26.** *Subluxation of the big knuckles; can contribute to swan-neck deformity.*

(see page 100) that I could continue to use the protective position. Loss of ability to curl the fingers at the PIP joint means that the arthritic cannot grasp objects like flatware and may have to use utensils with built-up handles. I have not yet had to use these in my seventeen years of arthritis. I think this is remarkable, considering that fifteen years ago, before I exercised them properly, my fingers had started to become stiffened at wrong angles so that I could hardly grasp anything. The PIP joints of several fingers of my left hand were so far destroyed that the joint spaces practically disappeared as observed on the X ray. Joint space—the distance between the bones where they come together in the joint—is normally filled up by the cartilage which covers the ends of both bones. The cartilage is not seen in X rays because it does not contain the calcium of which bone is made and which is visualized in the X ray. Thus, when no joint space is seen, the cartilage must have disappeared.

I later developed ankyloses in several of the PIP joints. This can happen either by the bones growing together (bony ankylosis) or by fibers forming across the joint to stiffen it (fibrous ankylosis). The stiffness itself is disagreeable, as bumping into objects with the stiff finger is likely to produce pain. It is worse if the joint ankyloses at the wrong angle so that the finger becomes useless.

While the joints were still flexible, I had some functional splints made, the so-called swan-neck rings shown in figure 25 on page 88. (A functional splint is designed to allow you to perform tasks and not for complete immobilization.) The swan-neck rings are double rings connected at one point and made to fit snugly so that the finger is forced into as normal a position as possible. Wearing these rings, I was able to use my left hand for grasping because the middle phalanges were supported in the bend position and the distal phalanges could flex freely. Eventually, several PIP joints on the left hand ankylosed in a functional position and I did not have to wear the swan-neck rings anymore. My left hand remained functional, although in a limited way; some of the fingers are able to wrap around relatively large objects.

Metal swan-neck rings (preferable to plastic rings, since they are thin and therefore interfere less with grasping objects) usually are made in the orthotics departments of large hospitals or at rehabilitation institutes. Once the swan-neck deformity is fixed, with the phalanges stiffened at wrong angles, the only procedure I know of that makes such fingers less painful, and even useful to a limited extent, is joint-replacement surgery. Such surgery is available, using plastic implants in the joints. Some flexibility of joints is regained and, to a very limited degree, some strength as well.

## Boutonniere Deformity

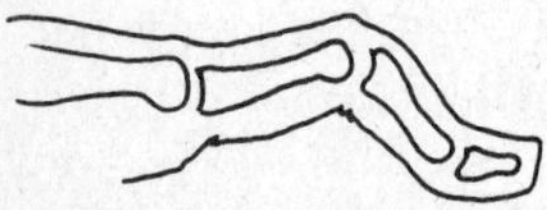

**27.** *Boutonniere deformity requires preventive splinting.*

This deformity (figure 27) causes the middle phalanx to become permanently flexed and the distal phalanx hyperextended. Objects cannot be gripped because of the bent position of the middle phalanx. This deformity comes about through damage to the tendinous structure on both sides of the PIP joint as a result of inflammation and swelling of the joint. A tear in this structure occurs which prevents the middle phalanx from being extended. The main therapy is prevention. The inflammation and swelling have to be combatted, mainly by resting the joint by immobilizing it in a short splint. The damage to the joint proceeds very slowly, and immobilizing it, which preferably should be done by an occupational therapist, is very effective.

One hand condition that I found very disabling although it is not a deformity is the inability to close your hand to make a complete fist. For instance, when I could not touch the palm of my hand with my fingertips, I had difficulty holding down the sleeve of a jacket when I put on an overcoat. Even such small disabilities produce great frustrations. I was gratified, then, to find out that after a week or two of daily finger-curling (see figure 37, page 100) my hand felt looser and that shortly thereafter I could again make a complete fist. I realized that I could overcome a progressive deforming process and keep the PIP joints flexible.

## HAND-REST SPLINTING

As I mentioned before, resting a joint helps to reduce the swelling and inflammation. The trouble with hands is that even if you rest "quietly" in bed, the phalanges of the fingers are still likely to move—for no apparent reason, or to pull up the bed cover, or to support your body when you roll over on your side. This is enough movement to prevent the joint from being sufficiently rested to reduce inflammation. Therefore, a rest splint is indicated if you want to reduce inflammation in all joints of the hands. Such a splint (see figure 23, page 85) gives complete rest to all finger joints as well as to the wrist. A molded plastic shell is available which can be adjusted to fit individual hands. It is individually fitted by an occupational therapist on prescription by a physician.

The hand-rest splint can be prepared by your occupational therapist so that only the proximal phalanges are supported and fingers can curl beyond the PIP joint. This is done when you have no problems with any of your PIP joints, and permits you some function in bed at night, moving the covers. If you have no problems with your thumbs, the thumb support can also be omitted. See figure 28. This is then classified as a functional splint. It supports the proximal phalanges in an extended posi-

**28.** *Functional splint supports the palm, keeps big knuckles in extension, front part of the fingers and thumb free to move.*

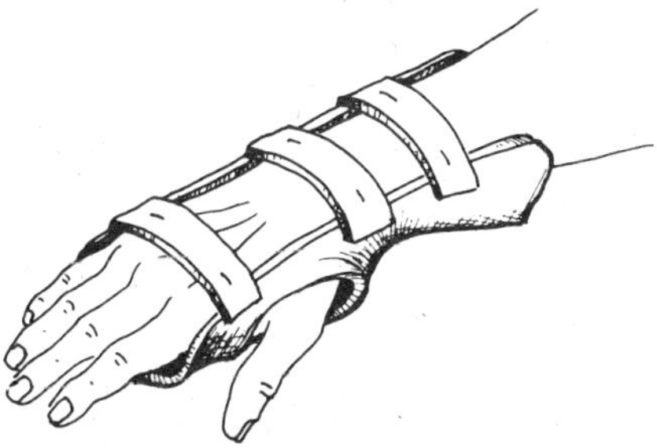

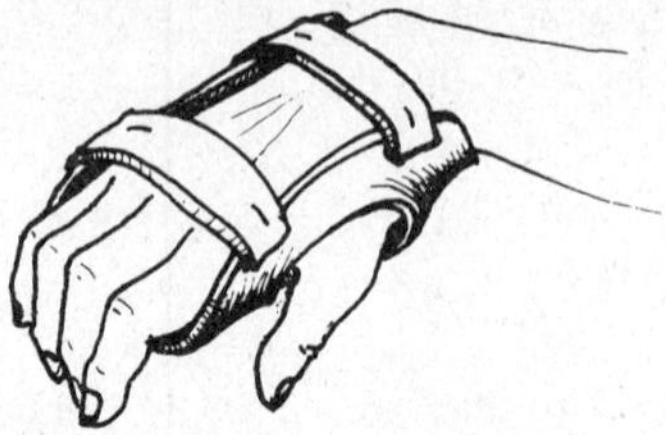

29. *The same splint without wrist support feels less clumsy.*

tion and prevents ulnar deviation. Figure 29 shows the same splint with wrist support removed, thereby providing better flexibility for the hand. Although the covered palm is somewhat clumsy, you will enjoy some hand function while wearing one of these splints.

I have found the use of these splints very beneficial, especially when worn at night during periods of high disease activity. When I wore the splint on one hand and not on the other, I could really notice the difference the next morning. When I consider that this simple mechanism means produced unswelling of my red, hot knuckles—something which twelve aspirin a day could not achieve and which cortisone injections into the joints could only temporarily achieve—I am very impressed by the performance of rest splints.

For reasons unknown to me, hand-rest splinting is not very popular, possibly because the rheumatologist, and especially the general practitioner, may be at a loss to advise you about where to get such a splint. I remember that after my rheumatologist told me to get one, I went through several frustrating experiences until I finally found a hospital with an occupational therapist who was geared to fit me with these splints. The therapist told me she had very little call for them.

## FUNCTIONAL SPLINTS

In addition to hand-rest splinting, there are also functional splints available in addition to the swan-neck ring described earlier, which I found to be the easiest of all the functional splints to tolerate. Another very useful splint is used to correct thumb deformity. In the usual thumb deformity, the proximal phalanx is bent and the distal phalanx is hyperextended to compensate for the flexed MCP joint. In this position your thumb can exert only a very small pinching force. Without splinting or surgical intervention, the thumb becomes useless.

I tried a variety of functional splints for my thumb which would keep the MCP joint in extension and permit flexion of the PIP joint. Most of them were very unpleasant to wear as they prevented rotation of the thumb to oppose the various fingers. After some research I found that the Warm Springs Foundation, Warm Springs, Georgia, had designed some slim metal splints which suited my condition and which permitted opposition of the thumb. To my surprise, I could not get this duplicated at any of the major rehabilitation and hospital centers in New York. Finally, the orthotics department of the Institute of Rehabilitation Medicine, New York University Medical Center, produced the design in plastic. I have worn this splint (figure 30) on my right hand now for approximately thirteen years. I wore a similar splint on my left hand for eight years and found to my delight that I could discontinue using it as the fibers around my MCP joint have regenerated in some way.

Splinting is worth trying for the thumb, but if it does not produce the desired result, there are some very sophisticated surgical procedures available in which tendons are rerouted across the MCP joints of the thumb to bring it back into extension again. It is advisable to look carefully for a surgeon who is experienced in this type of delicate surgery, however.

**30.** *Thumb splint helps straighten out zigzag deformity of the thumb.*

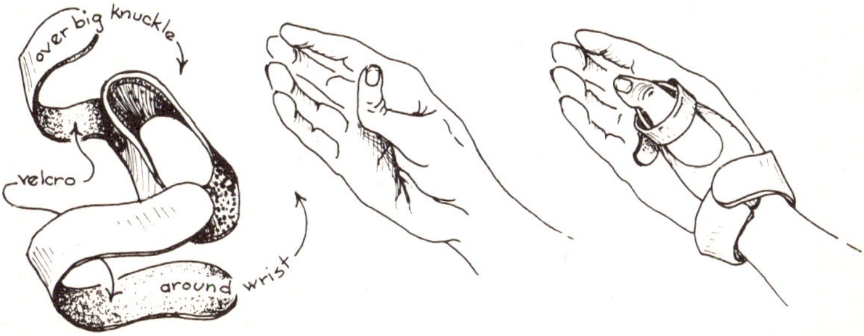

There are several other functional hand splints. Those designed to keep the proximal phalanges extended, or to prevent ulnar deviation of the fingers, are among the most useful. Several designs of such splints are known to occupational therapists (see figures 28 and 29 on page 91). It is very important to have these splints fitted individually; they tend to create pressure points around the large knuckles and to be clumsy, since they usually cover at least part of the palm. The prospect of being thus encumbered gives me a powerful incentive to exercise my fingers so as to delay the need for splinting. However, when hands are inflamed, such splints can be very useful in supporting the fingers in the correct position and preventing you from doing too much work and thereby increasing your discomfort.

## THE HAND GYM SYSTEM

We now turn to the exercises for the Hand Gym.* As I mentioned earlier, a clinical study of eighteen patients with rheumatoid arthritis and five patients with osteoarthritis produced statistically significant increases in strength and range of motion in those patients who had exercised twice a day for four months. Most patients reported improved function. A follow-up after four years showed that these patients had continued to exercise without supervision on the average of once a week—more than half of the rheumatoid arthritis patients had retained the improvement of function gained during the four-month study, and all of the osteoarthritis patients had maintained their functional improvements.

I noticed a definite improvement in my own function after about two weeks of exercising daily. I have been able to improve my handwriting at various times in the last fourteen years, when I was dissatisfied with it, by exercising several times daily for a few days.

The Hand Gym is supplied with a thirty-page instructional booklet and a large exercise chart with drawings and photographs as well as clear verbal descriptions of the exercises. The

* Cat. No. 1999 of Maddak Inc., available through selected surgical supply stores; or Arthritis Aids Division, price $20; (see Directory of Aids).

booklet contains a detailed description of seven range-of-motion exercises for the fingers and wrist and thirteen isometric strengthening exercises for the fingers, indicating also the anatomical names of the muscles.

The exercises are considered a highly efficient means of maintaining and increasing range of motion and strength—for arthritics as well as for persons without arthritis whose hands have stiffened with age, and for persons to whom manual dexterity is important, such as musicians, dentists, typists, and precision assemblers.

Persons with rheumatoid arthritis or an injury to the hand(s) require a balanced medical treatment program, of which the Hand Gym exercises form but one important part. The Hand Gym is an exercise aid; *no one with rheumatoid arthritis or an injury should use it without initial professional instruction and supervision by a physician or therapist.*

The stretching exercises Nos. 1, 3 and 4 help to increase and maintain the ranges of motion. The isometric exercises Nos. 2 and 5–14 provide strengthening of the hand muscles through the production of a *brief, maximal* effort of each muscle against resistance with the least amount of stress on the joints.

One five-minute session each day will help you regain or maintain agility and strength in your hands and fingers. Several sessions each day will help you regain elasticity of tightened muscles and develop endurance.

Please note also that gripping exercises should be avoided with those fingers that have excessive pain, joint swelling, or inflammatory tenderness in the second finger joints. This condition should be reported to your physician to enable further treatment and resumption of exercise.

Hand-Gym–type exercises can also be carried out without the Hand Gym (see page 106).

## THE DAILY FIVE-MINUTE WORKOUT WITH THE HAND GYM

To use the Hand Gym, hold it flat against your body at waist level with elbows against your sides, with the Hand Gym name facing upward. You may be sitting, standing, or lying down.

In the basic position for many exercises, rest your palms flat against the sides of the Hand Gym so that the roots of your fingers lie against the foam cushions. Insert your fingers into the proper slots. Let your thumbs rest on the upper surface. Do each exercise with both hands simultaneously.

To help prevent finger deformities and minimize pain, the "protective position" for the rheumatoid hand is used (figure 31).

- Fingers should be slightly spread, large knuckle joint should be kept straight, and small joints should be bent slightly.
- When you are holding the Hand Gym as described above, your fingers are supported in this position. Joints are properly lined up, and pain is minimized. According to present medical opinion, deformities can be prevented or reduced if the hand is held in this "protective position" during exercises and when grasping things in daily activities.
- In closing your hand when grasping, it is harmful, due to the disease, to bend the big knuckle joint since this puts stress on that joint and contributes to deforming the hand by stretching the ligaments. Use of the Hand Gym encourages the correct position.

If there is swelling or pain in the middle joint of any finger, omit exercises for this finger until it is improved. Consult your doctor.

## THE EXERCISES

### 1. Finger Spreading Without Resistance

If your hands are normal do this without the Hand Gym. However, if you have arthritis or another hand problem, use the Hand Gym for support. Rest your palms against the Gym and leave your fingers "floating" free outside the slots (figure 32).

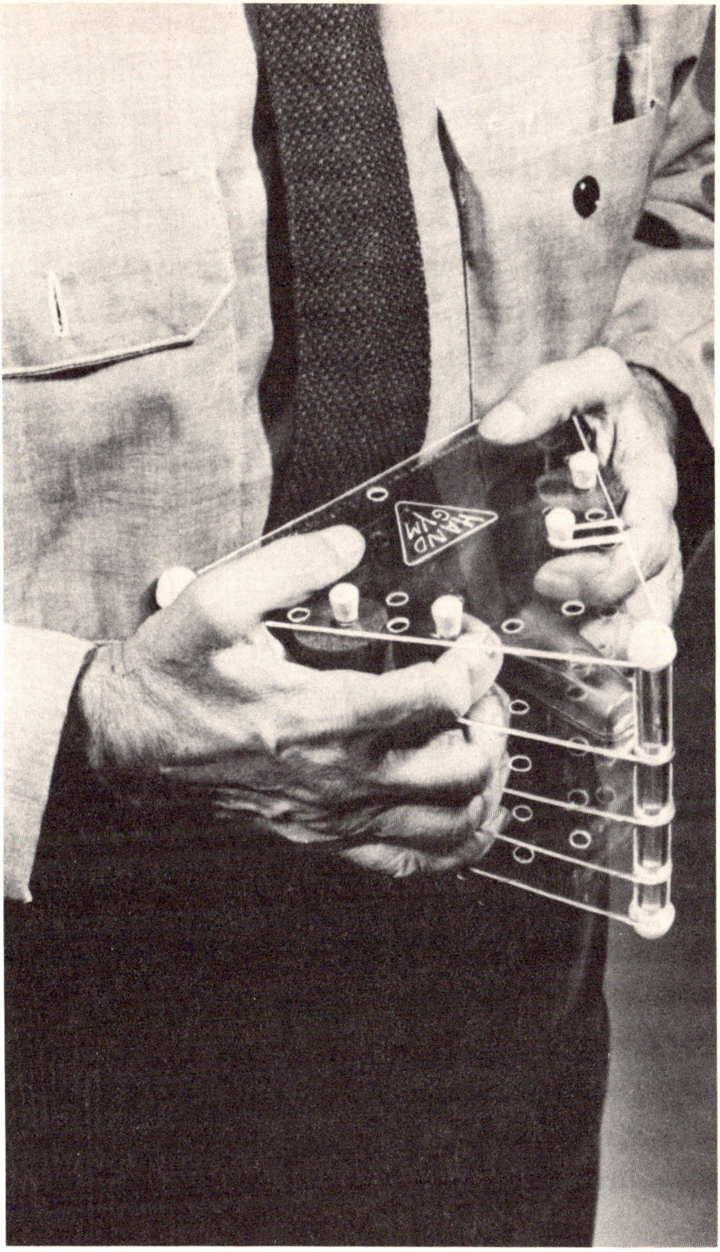

**31.** *Exercising with the Hand Gym. Fingers in "protective position."*

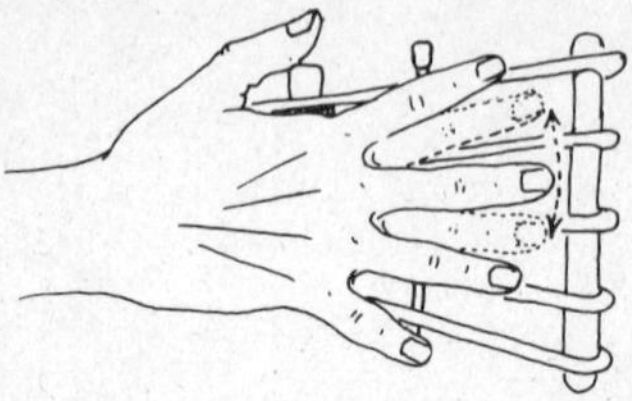

**32.** *Finger spreading without resistance (with or without Gym).*

Spread fingers as far apart as you can, then press them tightly together. Repeat four times. Now spread fingers apart and move middle finger up toward index finger, and then down toward ring finger. Repeat four times.

Be sure that you do not omit moving the middle finger—separately—toward the index finger and again toward the ring finger. This may not be easy at first, but you will succeed after a while. I have observed that with many people—even musicians, whose hands could be expected to be very nimble—the middle finger is the first one to exhibit stiffness.

If you require support for your fingers in order to flatten the hand, and you want to do it in the course of the day when you do not have the Hand Gym available, you may perform the exercise while pressing the palms of your hands near the roots of your fingers against the edge of a table.

## 2. Finger Spreading With Resistance

Hold the Hand Gym in the basic position, but let fingers rest against exercise bar (in second hole above foam cushions).

Spread fingers apart, pressing outward against walls of Hand Gym as hard as possible (figure 33); hold to a count of 6. Now bring fingers together, pressing as hard as possible inward against walls (figure 34); hold to a count of 6. Press middle finger against one wall and hold to a count of 6; then press it against opposite wall and hold to a count of 6 (figure 35). Then do the same with each of the other fingers.

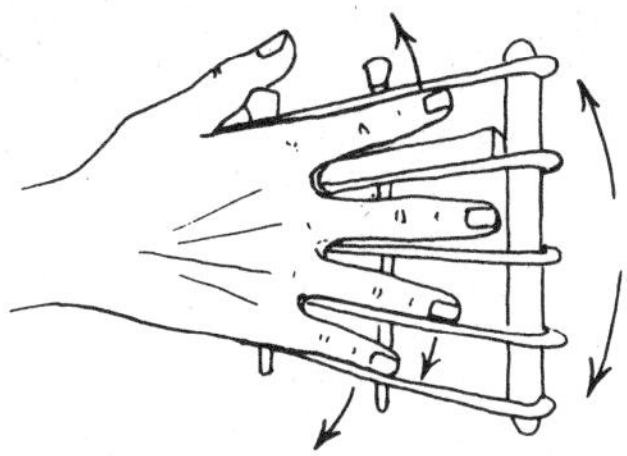

**33.** *Spread fingers forcefully outward against the walls of the Gym for a count of 6.*

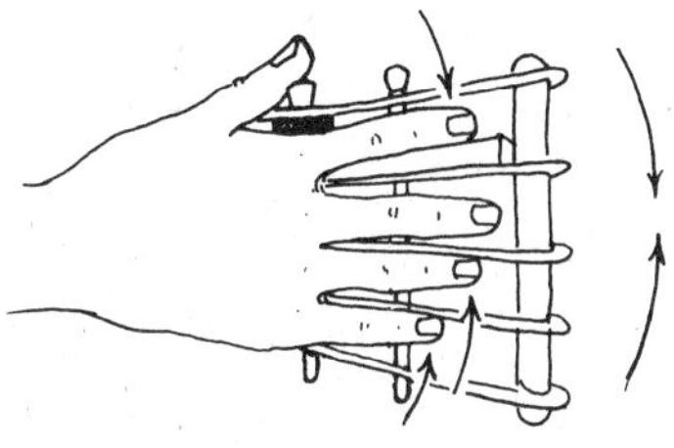

**34.** *Bring fingers together against the walls of the Gym forcefully for the count of 6.*

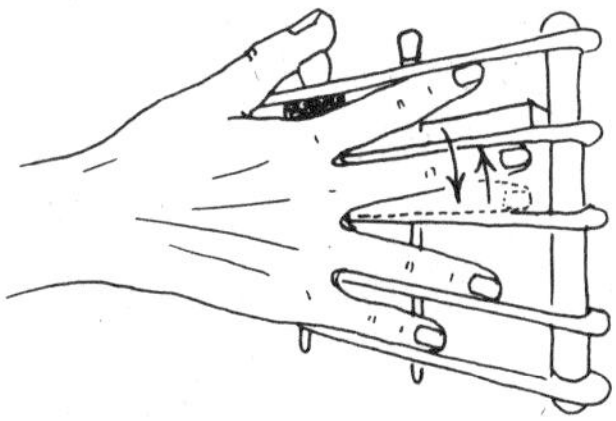

**35.** *Press middle finger, first strongly, against one wall for a count of 6, then against the opposite wall.*

This, together with finger curling with resistance, is one of the most important exercises on the Hand Gym. The Hand Gym structure works here to advantage, and cannot be easily replaced by other objects in the household. When you place your fingers into the slots and spread them against the walls, you will become aware of the strength with which each finger can press against the one side or the other side. You will then also notice, by comparison, that some fingers may be weaker than others, especially when pushed in one or the other direction. This should give you an incentive to exercise the weaker finger(s) diligently in order to achieve a good balance of strength. The abduction and adduction of the fingers are accomplished by the interossei which help rotate the finger, as when grasping a pencil, an eating utensil, or a hammer.

## 3. Finger Curling Without Resistance

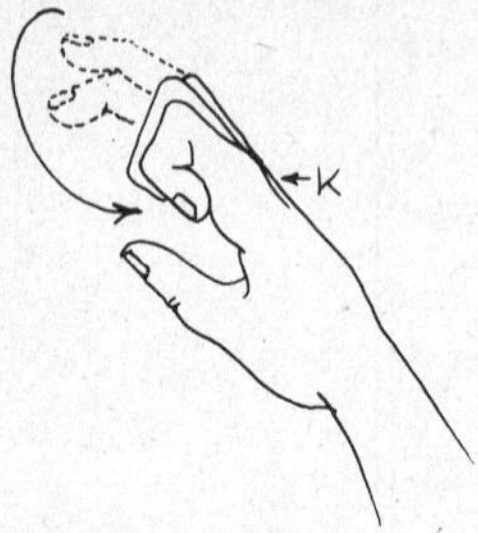


36. *Start with fingers straight. Slowly curl fingers, keeping large knuckles "K" straight, 4 times briefly. If you cannot touch fingertips to palm with large knuckles straight, practice next exercise with the Hand Gym.*

If your hands are normal, do this without the Hand Gym (figure 36). However, if you have arthritis or another hand problem, use the Hand Gym for support.

Start with fingers straight. Then curl fingers into a hook; it is very important to keep knuckle joint "K" straight while doing this. Continue curling as hard as possible until fingertips touch palms. Repeat four times.

This exercise tests your flexibility. The arthritic often will require the support of the Hand Gym and usually will not be able to touch the palm with the fingertip while keeping the big knuckle (MCP) straight.

## 4. Finger Curling With Resistance

Hook fingers around foam cushions and squeeze briefly four times, as hard as possible each time, *keeping knuckle joint "K" straight*. (Figure 37.)

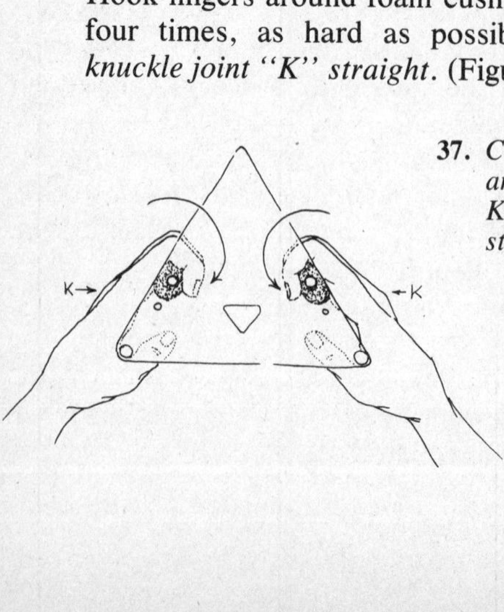


37. *Curl fingers forcefully around foam rubber 4 times. Keep big knuckles "K" straight.*

This is a very important exercise to keep the fingers flexible and to loosen the intrinsic muscles and thereby counteract the very disabling swan-neck deformity. Squeezing briefly four times should not produce any pain. If it does, or if the middle (PIP) joint of the fingers is inflamed, swollen, or painful, omit this exercise until the finger is recovered. Consult your physician.

## 5. Finger Straightening With Resistance

Place exercise bars in second holes above cushions, away from the edge, and stretch rubber bands across the ends of the bar as shown in illustration.

A. Insert fingers in slots between rubber band and exercise bar so that rubber band is stretched across lower part of fingers above big knuckle joints (figure 38). Push each finger (the same finger of each hand at the same time) as hard as possible outward against the rubber band. Hold to a count of 6 each time.

B. Pull fingers out far enough so that upper part of fingers rest against the rubber band. Then push each finger outward against the rubber band, as hard as possible. Do this with one finger of each hand at a time. Hold to a count of 6 each time. (Figure 39.)

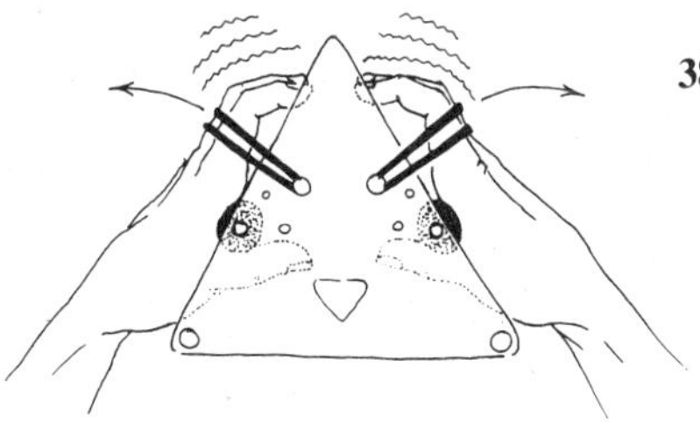

**38.** *Push fingers of both hands outward against rubber band and hold to a count of 6. If possible, exercise each finger separately.*

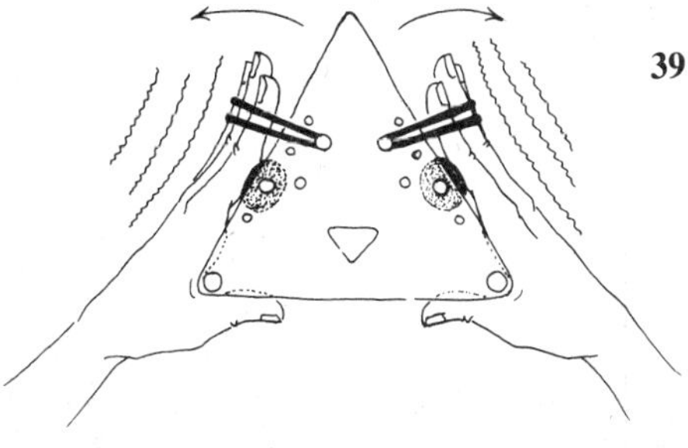

**39.** *Slip hands down so middle joint rests on foam rubber. Push forefinger out against rubber band for a count of 6. If you can, exercise each finger separately.*

The extrinsic extensor muscle, which helps to keep fingers straight and acts together with the interossei to rotate the fingers, is strengthened in A.

In B, the lumbricalis muscle is strengthened. This muscle helps to straighten the forepart of each finger and helps to control the pinch between tips of fingers and thumb. It also controls the strength of tapping, such as in typing or piano playing, by acting as a break on the profundus muscle which bends the fingertip.

## 6. Finger Bending, Distal Phalanx

Place exercise bar in second hole above foam cushions, away from edge, and stretch rubber band across ends of bar, as shown in illustration (figure 40).

Place fingers in slots just far enough so that fingertips can rest on bar. Keeping knuckle joint "K" straight, press each finger near the *tip* one at a time against the bar as hard as possible. Hold to a count of 6 each time.

This exercise strengthens the profundus muscle, which is located in the forearm and sends its tendon all the way out to the fingertip to bend it. This exercise, as well as the next one, is safe for the rheumatoid arthritic to use only if he can flatten out his hand so that the MCP joint, big knuckle "K", is kept straight during the exercise. I recommend that persons who cannot flatten their hands against the top of the bed not use the Hand Gym, since they will be unable to assume the protective position which safeguards the big knuckle during exercises. They should work with a therapist to loosen their hands first, if possible, and to straighten them sufficiently to fit the Hand Gym.

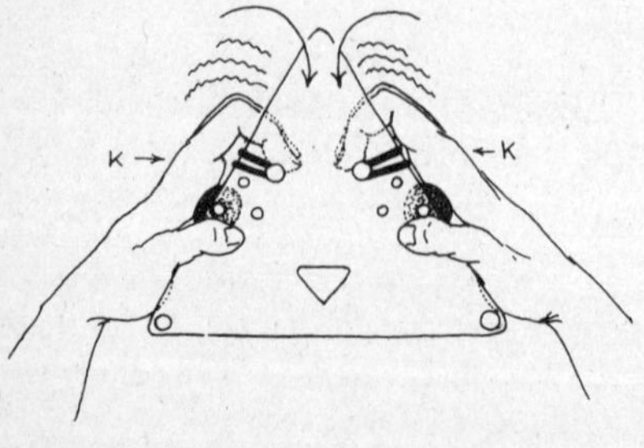


**40.** *Press fingers near the tip, one at a time, against the bar as hard as possible, each for a count of 6 (large knuckle "K" straight).*

## 7. Finger Bending, Middle Phalanx

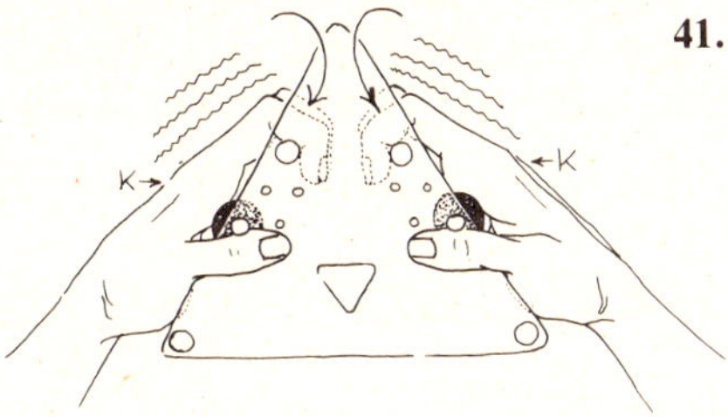


**41.** *Press middle section of each finger, one at a time, against the bar as hard as possible, for a count of 6. (Note that bar is moved for this exercise to second hole above foam rubber. Again, large knuckle "K" straight.)*

Place exercise bar in second hole above foam cushions, close to the edge.

Press *middle* section of each finger, one at a time, against the bar *as hard as possible.* Hold to count of 6 each time. Remember to keep knuckle joint "K" straight (figure 41).

This exercise strengthens the sublimis (also called superficialis) muscle, which is also located in the forearm and whose tendon leads into the hand to bend the middle joint (PIP) of the fingers. This is the principal muscle used in carrying such heavy loads as suitcases or in gripping tightly, as around the handle of a hammer.

## 8. Sideways Thumb Movement (Up)

Pull each cushioned hand-rest bar out one-half inch. Holding the Hand Gym in the basic position, push thumbs up against the protruding bars as hard as possible; hold to a count of 6 (figure 42).

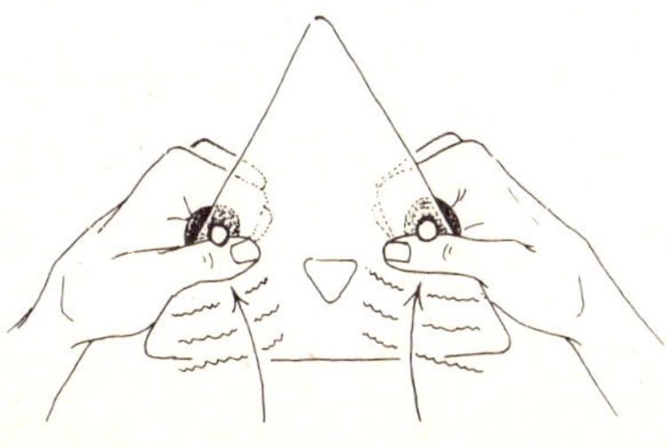

**42.** *Pull exercise bar out a little. Press thumbs forcefully* up *against bar to the count of 6.*

### 9. Sideways Thumb Movement (Down)

Keep cushioned hand-rest bars pulled out one-half inch. Press thumbs *down* as hard as possible against protruding bars, as illustrated (figure 43). Hold to a count of 6.

### 10. Thumb Flexing (With Thumb Straight)

Keeping thumbs *straight,* push in against the ends of the hand rest bars with each thumb, as hard as possible (figure 44). Continue pushing and hold to a count of six.

### 11. Flexing, Tip of Thumb

Hold the Hand Gym in the basic position. Press the *tip* of each thumb as hard as possible against the outside wall (figure 45); hold to a count of six.

### 12. Thumb Straightening, Proximal Phalanx

Curl the fingers of your left hand around the top of the Hand Gym. Place left thumb between first and second walls. Now bend thumb at small joint, pressing the *joint* as hard as possible against front wall (figure 46). Hold to a count of 6. Repeat with right thumb.

### 13. Thumb Straightening, Distal Phalanx

Proceed as in last exercise, but this time press the *nail* of each thumb against the outside wall as hard as possible (figure 47). Hold to a count of 6 each time.

### 14. Thumb Rotation

With index fingers and thumbs lying flat on outer wall, ''roll'' your thumbs along the surface of the wall toward you, then press them against wall as hard as possible (figure 48). Hold to a count of 6. If you prefer, do this one thumb at a time.

The last seven exercises show various directions in which the thumb is pressed up and down, flexed and extended, and finally rotated. Individual muscles usually are responsible for obtain-

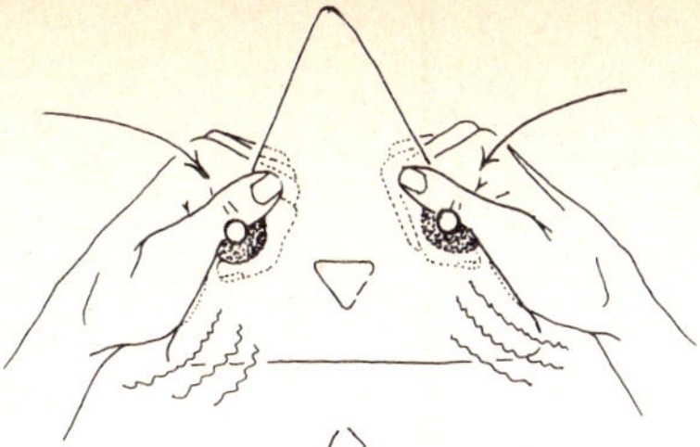

**43.** *Press thumbs forcefully* down *against exercise bar for a count of 6.*

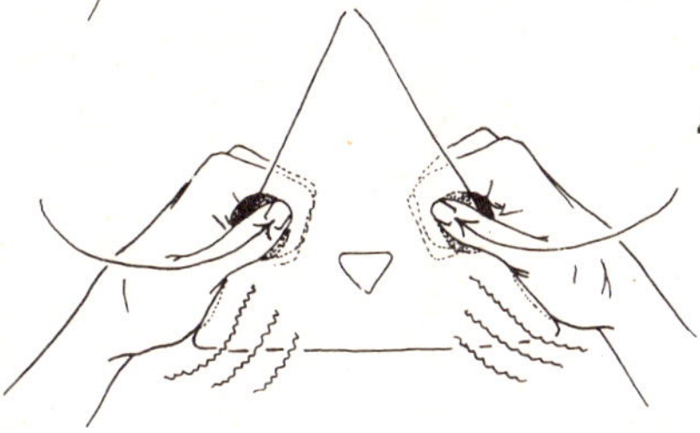

**44.** *With straight thumbs, press against bar ends firmly for a count of 6.*

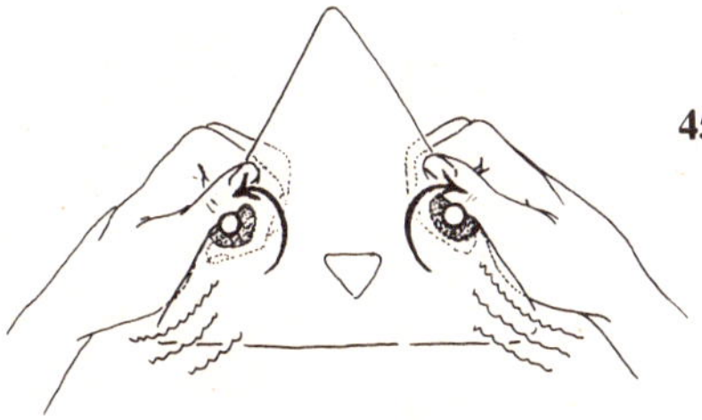

**45.** *Press tips of flexed thumbs firmly against outside wall of Hand Gym.*

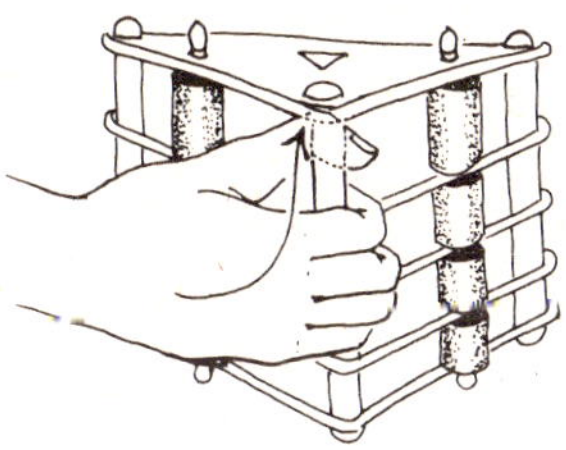

**46.** *Press thumb joint outward against Hand Gym's inner frontwall. Hold for a count of 6. Repeat with other hand.*

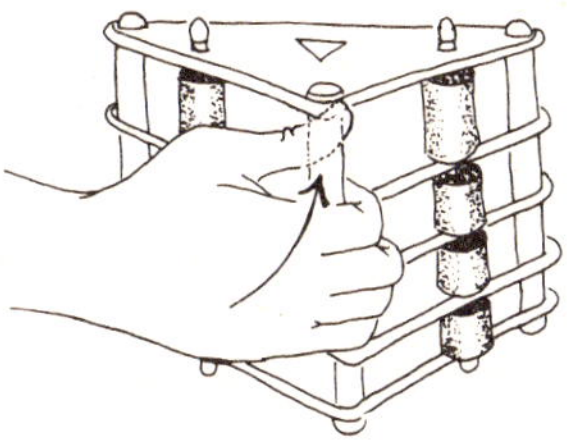

**47.** *Assume the same hand position, but press the thumbnail outward for a count of 6.*

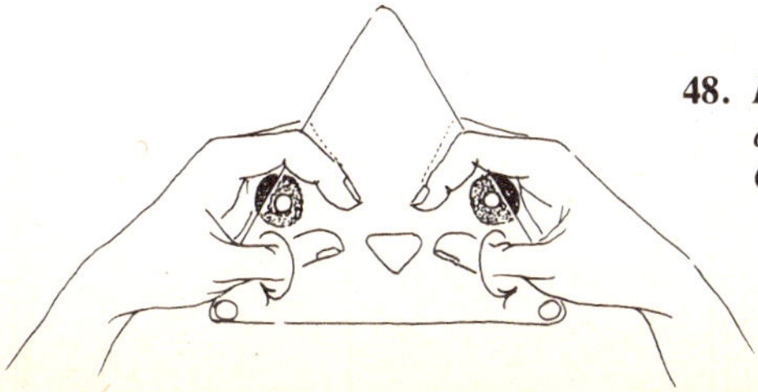

**48.** *Press outer side of thumbs against the front wall of the Gym to the count of 6.*

ing these motions. The bellies of these muscles can be felt in the palm, near the root of the thumb, and form what is called the thenar eminence. As you give resistance to the thumb, you can notice contraction of muscles within the thenar eminence. When you give resistance to the tip of the little finger, you will notice contraction of the hypothenar eminence on the palm at the root of the little finger. A rotating, or opponens, muscle of the little finger, similar to that of the thumb, exists also and can be exercised as shown in the exercise booklet.

It is, obviously, important to keep the muscles of the thumb in shape. After all, it represents half the hand in grasping, as objects are grasped between this finger and the other four. If you require a splint to straighten out the MCP joint of your thumb, wear it during the exercises, since the Hand Gym does not supply support for the MCP joint of the thumb as it does for the other fingers. See figure 30, page 93.

After exercising for a few weeks, you will notice that as you grasp the thumb between the index finger and the thumb of the other hand and try to wiggle out of the pinch in various directions, your joints hurt less, being controlled now more by increased muscle power than by the ligaments, which may be weakened due to the disease and painful when stretched.

The last exercise, *Thumb Rotation,* is an isometric exercise to strengthen the opponens muscle of the thumb. However, it does not stretch the muscle; this is achieved to some degree by the first exercise. Specific stretching of the opponens muscle is accomplished by resting the hand on the table and lifting the thumb up as high as possible.

## EXERCISES WITHOUT HAND GYM

Exercises are shown carried out with the Hand Gym, mainly to clearly outline the protective position for the hand and directions of push and pull for the fingers. Using the Hand Gym should result in becoming accustomed to carrying over the protected hand position into daily life. Hopefully, with careful observation of the exercise diagrams, the exercises can be carried out even when a Hand Gym is not available. This is done by improvising various means of support for the underside of the

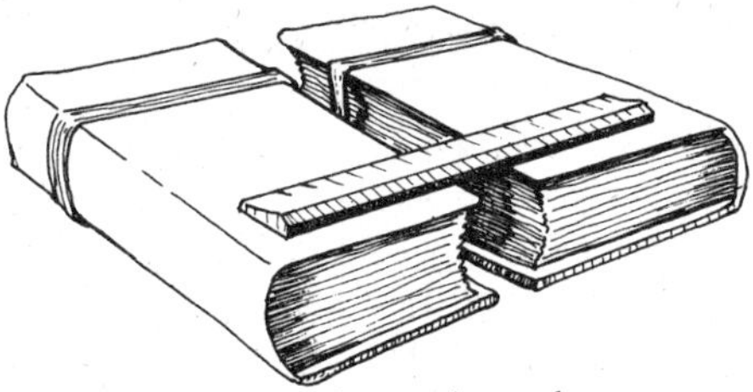

**49.** *Two books, rubber bands, and a ruler are arranged to provide support and guidance to the hand similar to that of the Hand Gym for some of the exercises.*

big knuckles and resistance for the various phalanges. For example, the hand can be pressed firmly against knee, fingers hanging loose; then press one fingertip at a time into the knee for a count of six (two to three seconds).

Pushing fingers sideways is more difficult to improvise without a Hand Gym. A dentist has devised a system, using two books arranged to create a slot—this enables exercise of one finger sideways at a time (figure 49). The underside of the knuckles rests on a ruler; the rubber bands are provided for extension exercises.

*Finger Curling With Resistance,* shown in figure 37, page 100, is difficult to do without the Hand Gym. You may curl fingers around foam rubber haircurlers pushed onto a pencil. Make sure that the big knuckles remain straight. This is difficult to achieve without some support for the hand. Use your ingenuity.

The Hand Gym is only an exercise frame which conveniently permits support for the hand and proper guidance for the fingers.

Other physical treatment considerations for the hand, besides exercises, include balanced activity to protect joints, heat and massage, and splints and gloves.

## PROTECTING THE JOINTS

Hands must always be used—if we can no longer use them, we are condemned to be helped even with eating, dressing, and body hygiene. I find it a very great incentive to avoid such handicaps. Therefore, it is of prime importance to maintain flexibility and sufficient strength to be able to operate within the limits of the condition dictated by the weakness of our joints. Even if you are able to handle a key or to open a screw jar, don't display false pride by unnecessarily performing these actions. Use a key holder and a jar opener to provide leverage. Use the protective position of the hand for grasping objects in daily life (see figure 14, page 81). Do not subject your hands to wear and tear; instead, maintain strength and flexibility through exercises. The daily stretching and the weekly strengthening exercise are probably sufficient to accomplish this—unless you have just passed through an acute phase and are weak, in which case you may require daily strengthening of finger muscles for a while. Remember that strengthening of the hands in the protective position with the Hand Gym is more efficient and less harmful than using your hands forcefully in activities like scrubbing and wringing laundry.

Use mechanical aids such as electric washers and dryers whenever you can. A booklet prepared by Judith Klinger with the Institute of Rehabilitation Medicine, New York University Medical Center, and the Campbell Soup Company, called *Mealtime Manual for People with Disabilities and the Aging,* contains a host of good suggestions and descriptions of gadgets that reduce the strain in the kitchen. The Arthritis Foundation also publishes a booklet describing useful self-help devices. Select and try some of them to help you in those activities which seem stressful for your hands.

## HEAT TREATMENTS

My rheumatologist suggested to me in the early stage of the disease to soak my hands for twenty minutes every morning in water as hot as I could stand, and after this to dry the hands and use an ointment (such as Ben-Gay) to lengthen the effect of increased circulation. Epsom salts can be added to the water for their beneficial effect on the skin.

This treatment has been beneficial at those times when I suffered from inflammation and pain in various knuckles of the hands. However, this "twenty-minute" bath can be quite time-

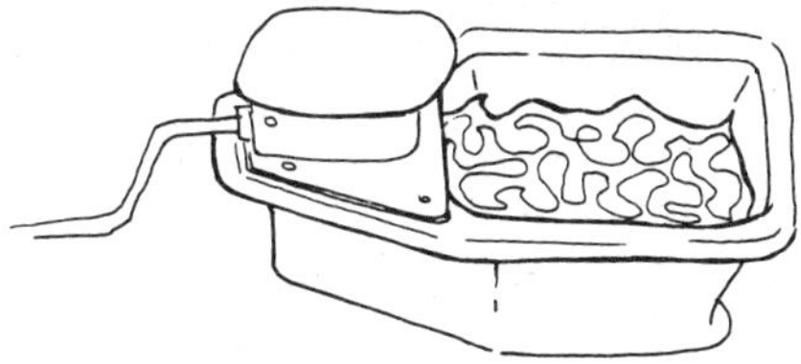

**50.** *A small Sears Roebuck whirlpool bath.*

consuming—it takes time to set it up, and you may need to rest afterwards. I found that water hot enough to increase the circulation in my hands to the degree that they turned red produced perspiration in other parts of the body. To save time, I started soaking my hands in a small whirlpool bath (figure 50) with very hot water for five minutes (see chapter 7, Hints and Aids). The massage produced by the water jet makes you more comfortable, permits the use of a higher water temperature, and helps in unswelling fingers slightly.

## SPLINTS AND GLOVES

Use of night rest splints or stretch gloves (see chapter 7) or even both at the same time, helps to reduce inflammation and swelling of the whole finger. I often feel so comfortable wearing these aids at night that I need only to wash my hands in soap and warm water in the morning to feel "in shape." Stretch gloves act like elastic bandages around each finger to force superfluous fluid out of them. They also cause the surface temperature to rise slightly, which is very pleasant. In the depths of winter, I wear a pair of fur-lined leather gloves. These keep my fingers warm and comfortable and also keep them in extension, though not quite as effectively as would a rest splint.

In chapter 5, What to Do About Pain and Stiffness, I describe two other treatment modalities for the hands—mudpacks and the paraffin wax dip. Both these treatments are supposed to provide a measure of relief from discomfort. I do not find them very effective for hands.

## STRENGTHENING THE WRISTS

Range-of-motion exercises for the wrists are shown in figures 16–20, pages 82–83. Strengthening of the wrists can be accomplished by following the motions of these exercises exactly, but with resistance furnished by the other hand or by pressing in the prescribed directions against some parts of your body—the knee, perhaps—or against a piece of furniture—perhaps a tabletop or the armrest of a chair.

## HAND AWARENESS

Once you have become accustomed to the various hand exercises and are aware of the function of various muscles, you may find it pleasant to incorporate some of the exercises into the motions of your daily life and to be aware of the stretching or strengthening these motions produce. For example, try several times a day to grasp a pencil between phalanges of your fingers with the MCP extended for a few seconds, as shown in figure 14, page 81.

At the slightest sign of developing tightness, or loss of range, or weakness, intensify your exercises by doing them more frequently. Clumsiness is not an inherent property—it can be largely cured by increasing the ranges of motion and strength of the fingers.

## DIRECTORY OF HAND AND FINGER SPLINTS

| |  |  |
|---|---|---|
| 1. | Wrist cock-up splint | figure 6, page 47 |
| 2. | Hand-rest splint | figure 23, page 85 |
| 3. | Swan-neck ring | figure 25, page 88 |
| 4. | Functional hand splint to control ulnar deviation | figure 28, page 91 |
| 4a. | Same splint as #4, but without wrist support | figure 29, page 92 |
| 5. | Thumb splint to control zigzag deformity | figure 30, page 93 |
| 6. | Outrigger splint used after joint implant surgery | figure 98, page 149 |

# 7
# Hints and Aids for Independent Living

Whenever I have experienced an acute phase of rheumatoid arthritis, I have had to rely on people to help me dress, eat, wash, open doors, or work in the kitchen. There is always that panic: will it blow over, will I be my able former self again? It does blow over, but after every acute phase we may lose a little flexibility and a little strength. Exercises will help us to maintain as much flexibility as possible. We have to be aware and work daily at it. Strength can also be increased with daily isometric exercises; however, we are limited in utilizing this added strength due to joint pain. Bad joint alignment, as the disease wreaks havoc with the ligaments, makes the joint less effective in transmitting the muscle power, and so our grip becomes weaker and weaker.

Functional splints can do wonders to keep joints in better alignment and improve our function. I have experienced that and described it earlier, with Swan-neck rings (figure 51) and a splint to correct the zigzag deformity of the thumb (figure 52). The functional splint shown in figure 53 prevents ulnar deviation and counteracts flexion contracture when wearing it. It permits only limited function, such as a hook grip. In figure 54 without wrist support, the splint feels less clumsy. But all we arthritics and, even more generally, old people, will start to experience difficulties in functions such as zipping the back zipper up, opening jars, buttoning the top button on a shirt, getting up from low chairs, etc. Don't despair—there is hope. There are many helpful hints on how to make things easier for yourself, and

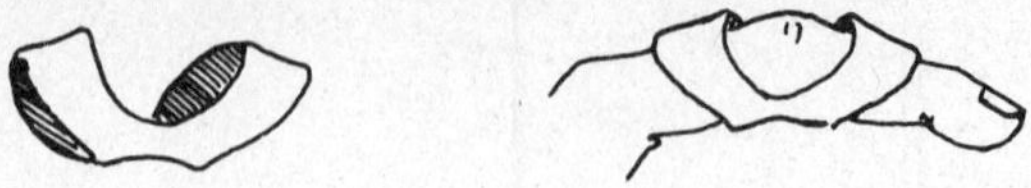

**51.** *Swan-neck deformity.*

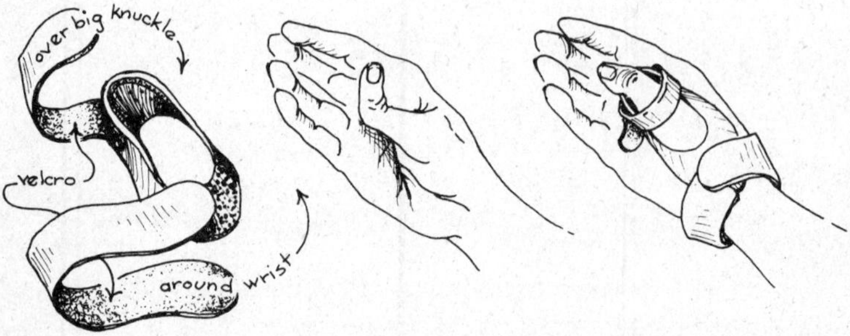


**52.** *Thumb splint helps straighten out zigzag deformity of the thumb.*

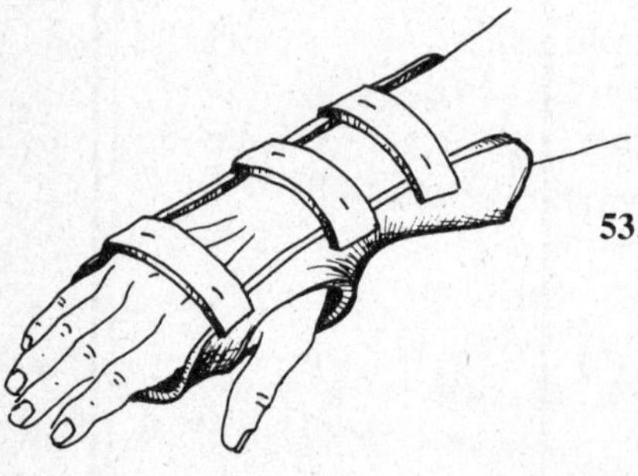

**53.** *Functional splint supports the palm, keeps big knuckles in extension, front part of the fingers and thumb free to move.*

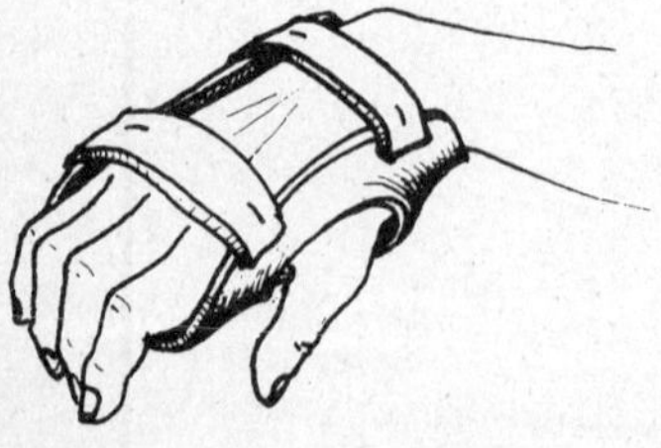

**54.** *The same splint shown in Figure 53, but without wrist support, feels less clumsy.*

mechanical devices which can help you continue to do things independently. The ingenuity of many inventive people from many lands has created a number of these aids. There are Canadian, Swedish, German, Italian, and English aids in addition to all the ones made in the U.S.A. that are ready to help you.

How to obtain the best hints and aids? That's the question. It is the job of the occupational therapist, if one is available, to help you. Your doctor can refer you to one. There are Arthritis Clubs where patients share the information that is available. It is not easy to obtain such information; although there are hundreds of manufacturers and distributors around, some handle only one or two items. The Arthritis Foundation has a book available listing hundreds of aids and sources, and may also have a display of aids. Sometimes too much information may be as bad as too little, and it is frustrating to get an answer from a manufacturer or distributor announcing that a desired item has been discontinued. Your local surgical or medical supply dealer may be of help looking through his catalogues together with you. I am going to share with you the awareness necessary to help yourself, information on aids you can make yourself and those you can buy, and the sources that supply them (see Directory of Aids).

You will be surprised that in a book about hands, I will tell you about raised toilet seats. Well, medical opinion states that the arthritic should preferably not use his hands to push off when getting up from a seated position, to prevent enhancing the development of hand deformities due to stress.

I am using or have tried practically all the aids I describe. Due to exercises with the Hand Gym, I believe, my fingers have remained sufficiently flexible so that I do not have to use "built up" handles for cutlery and various utensils. Try to keep as flexible as possible by exercising daily; you can guide utensils with better precision without the use of built up handles. But for those who need them, I will present the best hints and aids I know of.

Now let me give you some hints and tell you about some mechanical aids to keep you independent of others in your daily life. You certainly will not require all the advice given or all the aids presented. Maybe your major problems have not been addressed, but I hope you will find something new and useful for you here. Here we go!

## GETTING OUT OF BED

- When you are ready to get out of bed, first sit at the edge of the bed with legs dangling down. Now bend forward as you get up. Do *not* get up sideways. This may strain (wrench) your lower back with resultant pain which may prove hard to get rid of.
- Try not to use your hands to "push off" as you get up from your bed. If absolutely necessary, push off with the heels of your hands, letting your fingers dangle over the edge of the bed. Consider raising your bed. Try out the best height for you. You may use bricks as a temporary support. Each brick is two inches (5 cm) thick. Three bricks (six inches [15 cm]) under each leg may be sufficient. You should be able to step out of bed easily without support by your hands. A carpenter will be able to attach legs of the selected heights for you (figure 55). You will find a description of how to construct such legs in *Aids and Adaptations* from the Canadian Arthritis and Rheumatism Society, 45 Charles St. E., Toronto M4Y 153, Canada ($2.50). I have never come across any reliable ready-made, commercially available leg extenders for beds or chairs.

## IN THE BATHROOM

- Should you have difficulties in getting up from the toilet without getting help from somebody or straining your hands holding on to a bar or a nearby hamper, don't despair. You are one of millions of people who have this difficulty and you can be helped with a raised toilet seat. They are doughnut-shaped, easily place on and removed from the toilet bowl. See figure 56. There are two models available: one for four-inch (10 cm) elevation of the seating heights, and one for six-inch (15 cm) elevation. The 4″ one weighs three pounds (1.4 kg), the 6″ one four and a half pounds (2 kg.). This is something to consider.

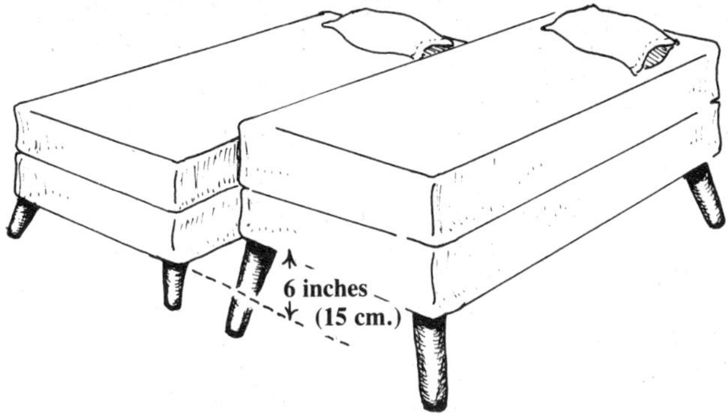


**55.** *If you have difficulty rising from your bed without pushing off strongly with your hands, install longer bed legs. 6" (15 cm) higher legs may be just right.*

See Directory of Aids for further information. For your comfort in getting up, the right size is important. You may experiment by piling a four-inch (10 cm) thickness of telephone books on top of the cover of the toilet and see how easily you can get up. If this is not sufficient for your comfort, choose six inches (15 cm).

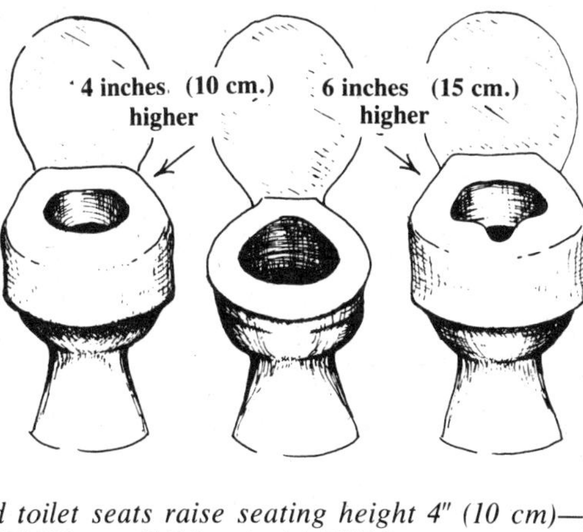


**56.** *Elevated toilet seats raise seating height 4" (10 cm)—AA 72580, (SR) 8AH1186—or 6" (15 cm). AA 72586*

- Now to the sink. Use your left hand to open the water taps (counterclockwise motion), and your right hand to close them (clockwise motion). This way your fingers will always move in a direction opposite to ulnar deviation, avoiding encouragement of this type of deformity.
- Should you have difficulties turning the taps limited by knuckle pain, ask your plumber whether he can install fluted conical plastic tap handles (figure 57).
- An alternative to the above is a tap turner aid (figure 58); see Directory of Aids. This aid easily engages conventional cross-head handles. The handle is seven inches (18 cm) long, thereby increasing leverage to open the tap easily.
- I use a small plastic or paper cup for holding water to rinse my teeth. Avoid regular glasses; they are heavy to hold and make a mess when they break due to clumsy handling.
- The thin toothbrush handle may present a problem for you if your fingers have become too stiff to close around it for a proper grip. This brings us to the general subject of built-up handles. There are various ways to provide a large diameter handle for easier grip. One way is to slip the pink foam rubber part of haircurlers over the handles (figure 59). These come in various diameters and are rather soft, and therefore collapse to a small diameter. A somewhat larger diameter can be obtained by using the round dark grey foam cushions of the Hand Gym (figure 60). These are available in the reasonably priced replacement part set for the Hand Gym (see Directory of Aids). You get eight cylindrical cushions, enough for building up two handles.
- A larger diameter build-up, and a more solid consistency, is achieved by using a bicycle handle. Such replacement handles are available wherever bicycles are sold. It is easy to insert your aid and fill up the handle with wood putty or another compound recommended by your hardware salesman. It is very much worth your while to learn the technique of building up handles yourself. You save money over buying ready-made devices, and in addition, you may slip a bicycle handle or foam rubber over the handles of devices which are commercially not available "built-up."

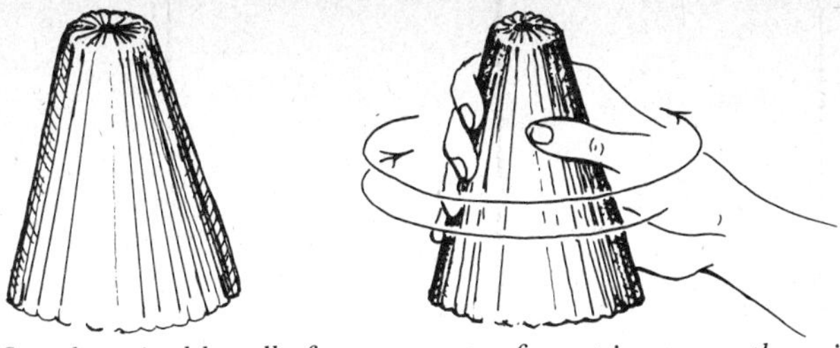

**57.** *A fluted conical handle for your water faucet improves the grip for the arthritic hand.*

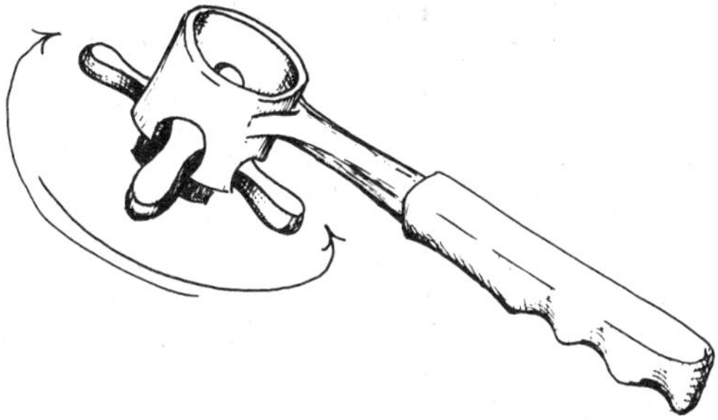

**58.** *Tap turner increases leverage to easily turn cross-head handles. AA 75315*

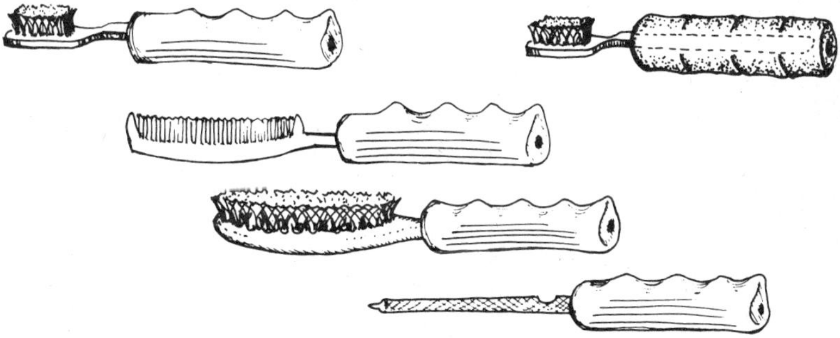

**59.** *Various grooming aids equipped with built-up handles: toothbrush, comb, nail file, and brush.*

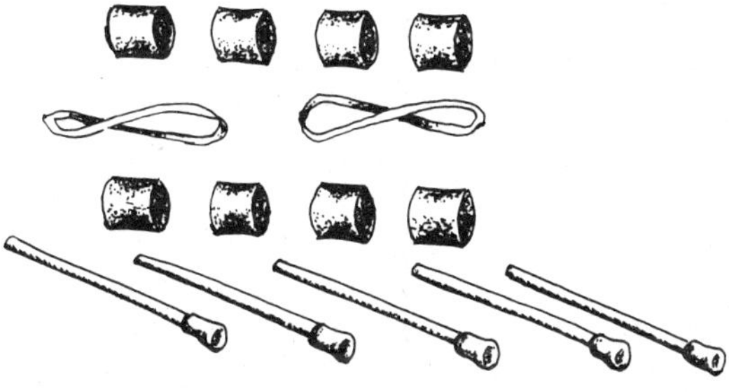

**60.** *The set of replacement parts for the Hand Gym consists of 5 exercise bars, 8 foam rubber cushions, and 2 rubber bands. AA 70902*

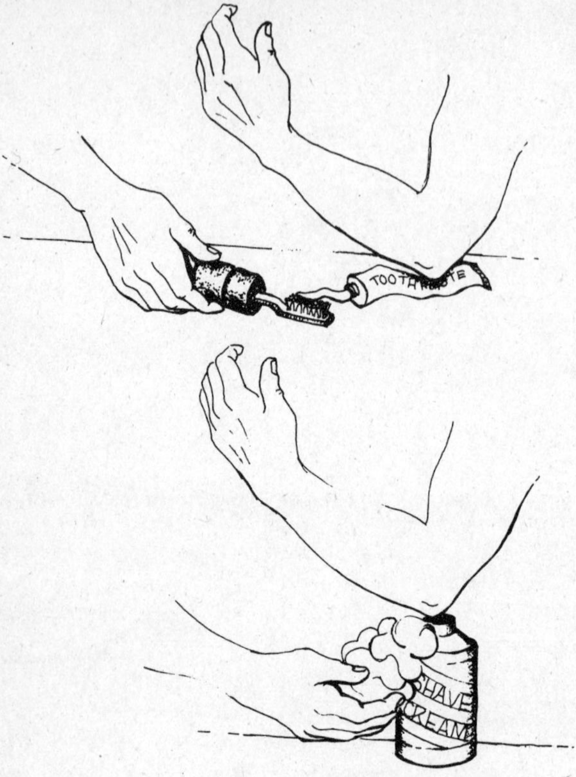


**61.** *Use the tip of your elbow to squeeze toothpaste from a tube or release shaving cream from a pressurized can.*

- If you have difficulty squeezing out toothpaste or shaving cream from the tube, use the tip of your elbow; do the same to release shaving cream from a pressurized can (figure 61).
- It is very difficult for arthritic fingers to apply dental floss. The dental floss holder shown in figure 62 is available to help you with this important dental hygiene. See Directory of Aids. You may want to build up the thin handle with foam rubber or a bicycle grip, if you have difficulty grasping it tightly.
- If it is difficult for you to use a nailbrush with your hand, get one that can be mounted with suction cups on your sink or counter top (figure 63). See Directory of Aids.

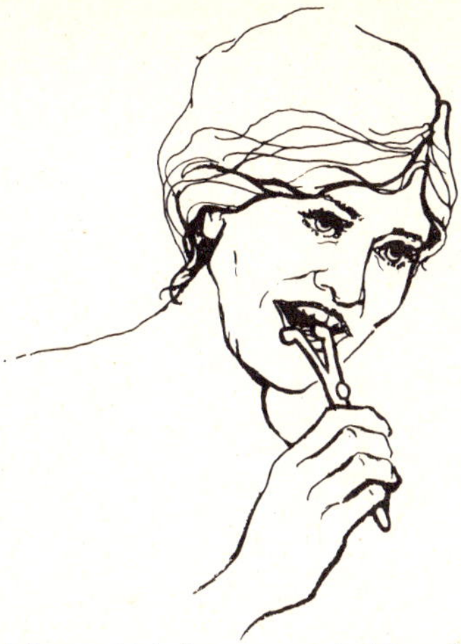

**62.** *The dental floss aid helps you to hold and apply dental floss without requiring great finger dexterity. AA 74155*

- Next we take a bath or a shower. A warm bath is preferable to dissipate stiffness. You need a good rubber mat in your bathtub so as not to slip. If you have problems getting into or out of the tub by yourself, you may be helped by grab-bars attached to the wall and/or rim of the tub. I highly recommend the advice of an occupational therapist for proper selection of the grab-bars and technique to get in and out of the tub to prevent needless accidents. Soap which has a loop of rope attached to it is available in drug stores. Hang it around your neck. Use a bath mitt. You can make yourself one by sewing two washcloths together after cutting them to fit the shape of

**63.** *Clean your fingernails with a nailbrush mounted by suction cups on sink. AA 74148*

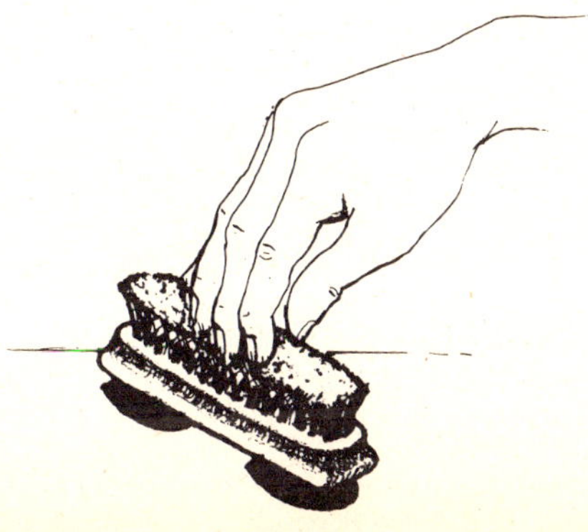

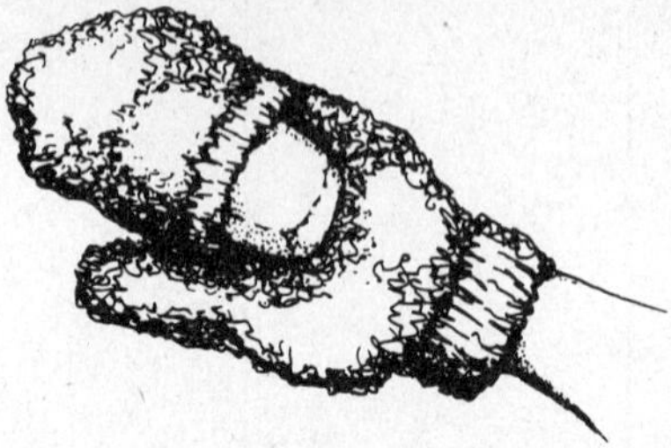

**64.** *Terrycloth wash mitt fits snugly around the wrist, with built-in elastic. It is equipped with a soap pocket. AA 74132*

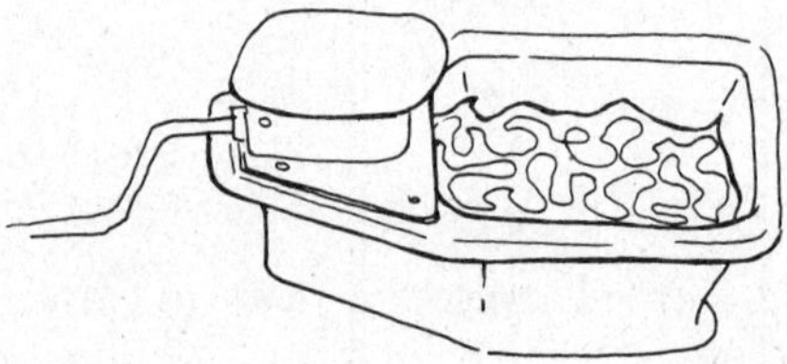

**65.** *Whirlpool bath permits you to use very hot water for better and longer-lasting relief. SR 8AH2262*

your hand. Or, if you prefer, you may buy one, as shown in figure 64 (see Directory of Aids). This one comes with a pocket for soap. A bathbrush with a long handle is helpful for reaching your back as well as your feet.

- Some people cannot get into or out of the bathtub, but can use a walk-in shower. Make use of a hand shower attachment to your showerhead. It might be useful to build up the handle with a bicycle grip.
- A hot whirlpool bath (figure 65) for hands is quite a rejuvenating experience.
- After your bath or shower, back to your bedroom—which should be comfortably warm so you don't get chilled during your limbering up routine, including the five-minute workout with the Hand Gym (figure 66); see Directory of Aids.

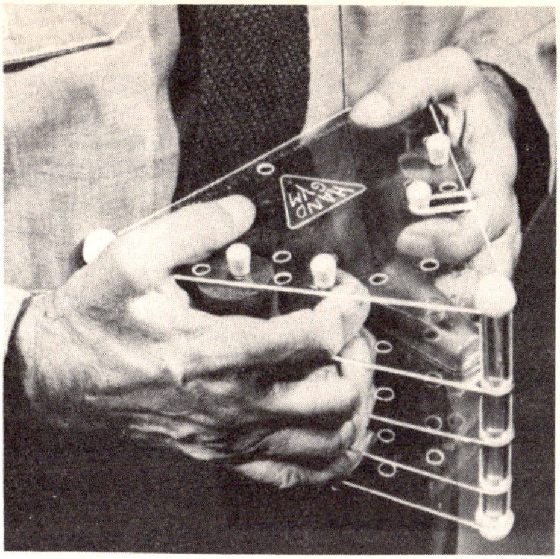


**66.** *The Hand Gym permits fingers to be exercised in all directions. AA 70900*

## GETTING DRESSED

- Dressing problems arise when you cannot easily reach down to your toes or over your shoulder to your back to the zipper closure. Reduced power for pinching the closure does not help, either. A number of aids can be very helpful. One, which can be called a "dressing stick," consists of a wooden stick with a hook at the end; it extends the reach of your hands. If you want to put on your underpants, you normally use both hands. If you cannot reach, you should have two dressing sticks to extend the range of both hands simultaneously. Figure 67 shows two designs for homemade dressing sticks. If you cannot make it yourself you can buy a twenty-inch (50 cm) dressing stick (see Directory of Aids). If you have difficulty reaching your zipper in the back, attach a little ring or loop to the zipper closure and operate it with the stick. The curved hanger would be especially useful for this. If you cannot pinch the zipper closure on your trousers properly to move it up and down, again insert a ring or loop and operate it with the hook of the dressing stick. If you have a hard time holding the stick, build up the handle with a bicycle grip. You can put on your trousers by inserting the hooks of two dressing sticks in the belt loops and pull. If you want to pull up underpants or slips, attach little loops to the underwear, insert the dressing stick hooks in the loops, and pull up.

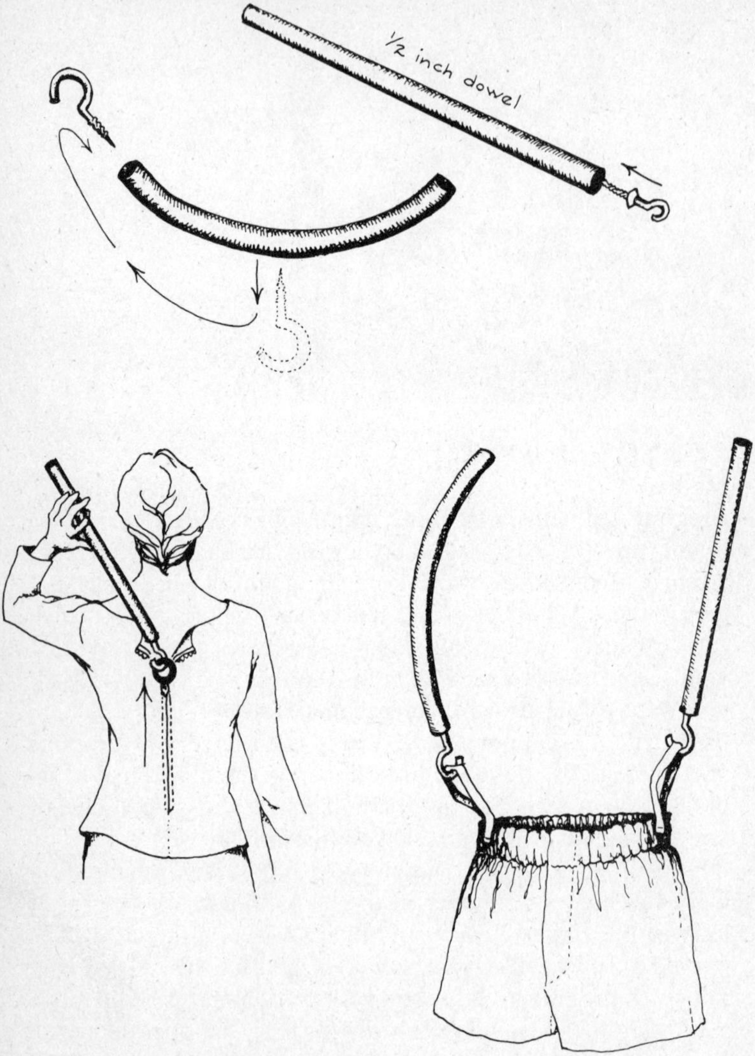


**67.** *A dressing stick helps extend the reach of your hands beyond your feet. AA 73881. A curved wooden hanger can easily reach over your shoulder. The hook can be a small cup hook, a larger hanger hook, or an in-between size. Attach tape loops to underwear and pull up with stick.*

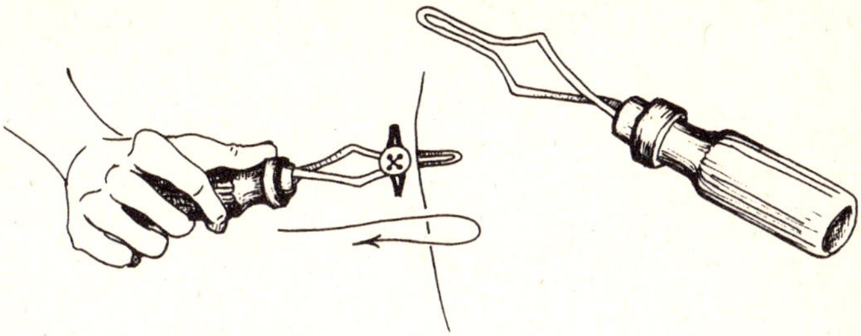

**68.** *A button loop may be used to handle small buttons. AA 73884*

- If you have difficulty handling small buttons, use a button loop (figure 68); see Directory of Aids.
- You can replace hard-to-reach buttons with Velcro pressure tape (figure 69). This tape can be bought in department and sewing supply stores. One strip of Velcro consists of thousands of little hooks that "mate" with thousands of little loops; when pressed together, they stick. They can be easily peeled apart again and reused without limit.

**69.** *Velcro tape can replace buttons in hard-to-reach places.*

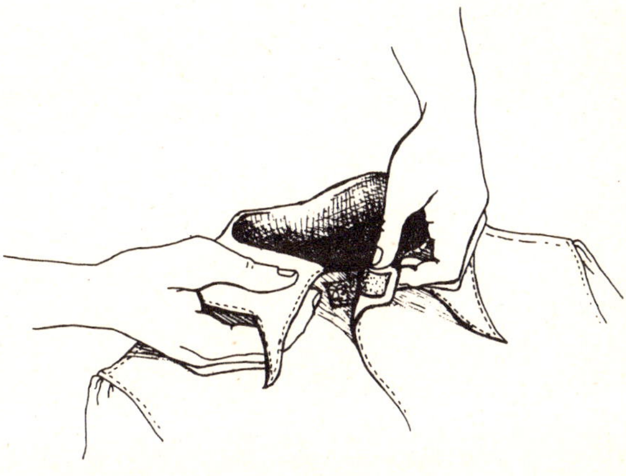

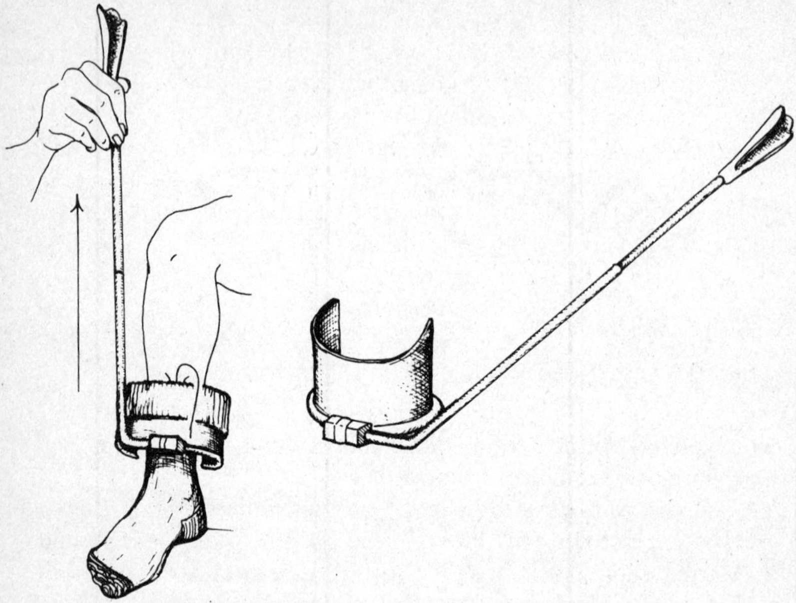

**70.** *The hose helper permits socks or stockings to be pulled over a plastic half cylinder. The foot is inserted and the hose is pulled up with the long handle. AA 73845*

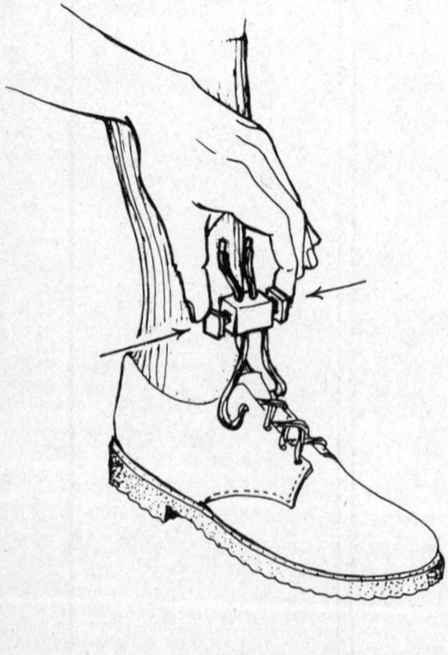

**71.** *A new device keeps regular shoelaces tight without tying them. AA 73810 & 73811. Extra length of laces is tucked into shoe top. A little button releases laces when desired.*

- Trying to put on or take off stockings as you slowly lose you ability to reach your toes is a nightmare. A most ingenious Italian device is illustrated in figure 70 (see Directory of Aids). Socks or stockings are pulled over a very smooth plastic half cylinder. The foot is fitted through opening thus created and by means of the long handle the hose is pulled over the foot. The end of the shoehorn, attached to the long handle, is shaped so as to easily remove the hose from the foot.
- A long shoehorn can be very useful. If you do not have a Hose Helper with an attached shoe horn and cannot locate one in local stores you can order a 17½-inch (44 cm) plastic model; see Directory of Aids.
- Elastic shoelaces permit shoes to be slipped on and off without tying or untying; see Directory of Aids.
- A remarkable new little device (figure 71) holds shoelaces tightly without tying; see Directory of Aids. The dressing stick (see figure 67) can be useful for loosening or tightening shoe-laces.

## KITCHEN ACTIVITIES

- In the kitchen, the first requirement is to have a chair from which you have no trouble getting up, and is easily moved about. Remember we talked before about the importance of elevated seating heights. I prefer a lightweight 24-inch (60 cm) high wooden barstool. You can attach glides for easier moving about. The 24-inch height is just right for working at a regular table or counter. A 30-inch (75 cm) high stool is still easier to get off from, but is a little too high for working or eating at a regular table, causing you to jam your legs and to stoop down too far (bad for your back). In a large elongated kitchen you may want two stools. A stepstool is just the right height and may substitute for one of the stools, but is more difficult to move. Try to arrange your pots and pans, cans, and cartons of supplies at an easy-to-reach level. Try to avoid having to bend down or reach too high up. Even with a reaching aid, things can fall down, hurting your hands. To learn in considerable detail how to arrange your kitchen consult the Mealtime Manual for People with Disabilities (see Directory of

Aids). If possible, consult an occupational therapist; they are experts in these matters. Often occupational therapy departments are equipped with model kitchens.

- How to open containers: Do not strain your fingers opening cartons; use a knife. To open a milk carton, use the heels of your hands rather than the thumbs to push back the flange (figure 72).
- Do not use a small hand-held can opener. Use a unit attached to the wall, with a large handle and gears. If you buy an electric can opener, get one which is fully automatic and makes the first cut with its own rather than your power. If you have to open sardine cans, do not use the small key furnished with them—unless you use a screwdriver through the opening of the key to increase leverage. It is best to use your usual can opener for even the sardine can if it will fit.
- Do not struggle with a jar top. Some people consider this a good exercise—I don't. There is a remarkable, reasonably priced jar opener called Un-Skru (figure 73); see Directory of Aids. It is mounted with screws to the underside of a shelf; it opens screwlids from three-eighths-inch (9.5 mm) diameter up to three and three-eighths-inch (8.6 cm) diameter. Use both hands to hold the jar.
- Get accustomed to holding most things in the kitchen with *both hands:* milk cartons, orange juice containers, pots and

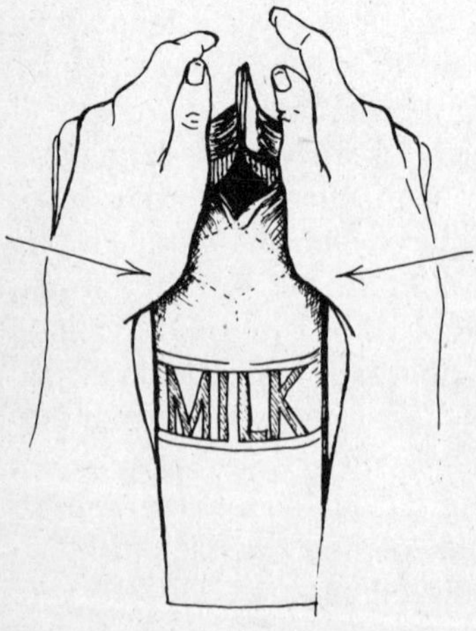


**72.** *Open a carton of milk with the heels of your hands. Save your thumbs.*

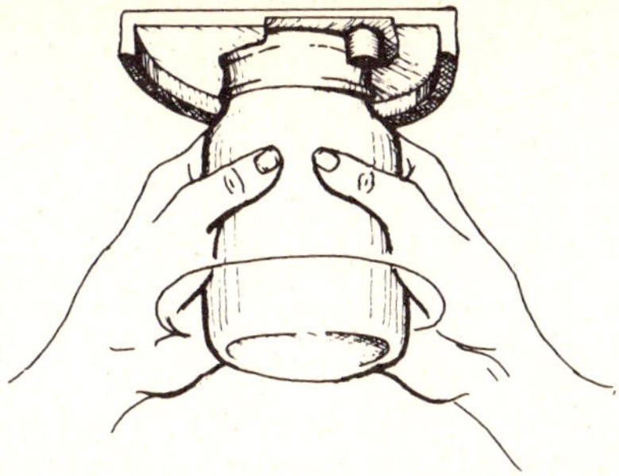

**73.** *The Un-Skru jar opener is extremely easy to use. Save your joints. Use both hands to hold jar. AA 75346, SR 8AH1366*

pans, bowls and dishes. If a pot has one handle, slip one hand underneath the handle; support the bottom of the pot on the opposite side with the other hand.

- Never *twist* your fingers around a handle of any tool in your kitchen like you would a pencil. Keep the line of MCP joints straight. If need be, build up handles to achieve this. Try to keep your MCP joints extended as much as possible. Remember the protective position of the hand from the last chapter. A new Swedish slicing knife (figure 74) has become available with a nine-inch (23 cm) serrated blade; see Directory of Aids. It is equipped with a saw-type handle, ideal in saving the knuckles from stress.

**74.** *A new Swedish slicing knife with 9″ (23 cm) serrated blade and saw-type handle to save your knuckles. AA 75326*

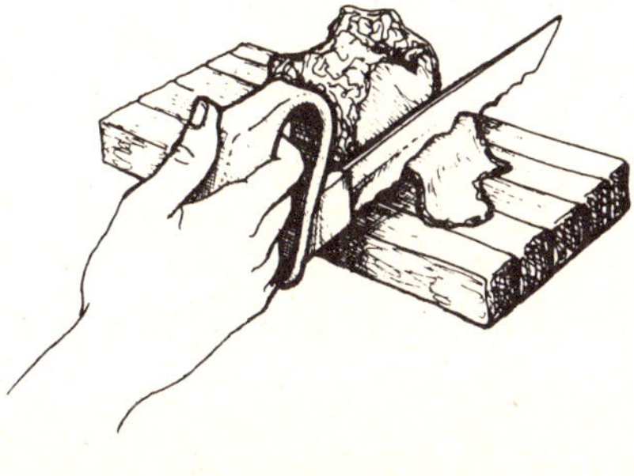

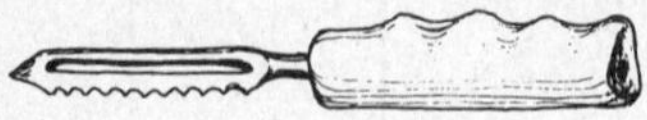

**75.** *Build up the handle of your potato peeler with a bicycle grip or buy the ready-made aid. AA 75330*

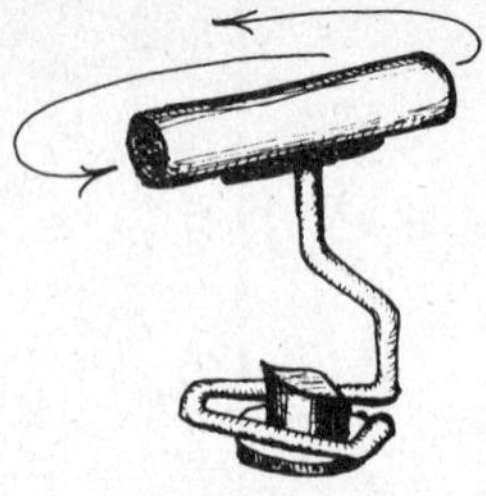

**76.** *A sturdy aid to turn knobs on stove and other larger knobs. AA75433*

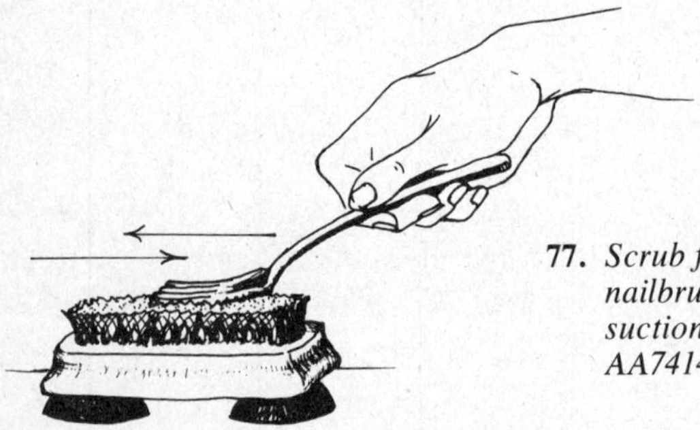

**77.** *Scrub forks and knives on nailbrush attached with suction cups to counter. AA74148*

- Some potato peelers may be hard on your knuckles. If your fingers have to curl around the thin handle, the peeling action transmits a strong twist to the knuckles. Build the handle up with a bicycle grip; or, if you prefer, buy the ready-made one illustrated in figure 75 (see Directory of Aids).
- This sturdy Swedish device (figure 76) helps you to open and close the often hard-to-turn controls of your stove. It may also be useful to turn other large knobs around the house.
- To help stabilize bowls and dishes, and even a cutting board, and prevent them from moving away as you use an electric beater and knives, you can place them on a piece of thin rubber sheeting obtainable from your drugstore. Two stainless steel nails driven through a wooden cutting board will help you to stabilize your piece of meat or head of lettuce on the board so that both hands are free for cutting.
- When you wash up, make sure not to curl your fingers when you use a sponge. Hold your hand down flat on it. You may curl the PIP and DIP joints, but hold the MCP joints straight.
- You can use a nailbrush, fastened to the counter top with suction cups, to scrub knives and forks (figure 77).

## EATING AND DRINKING

- Now we get down to the job of eating and drinking. Avoid teacups if you can. The extra long lever arm places big stress on the big knuckles. The smaller the diameter of a drinking cup, the better. Mostly people recommned using both hands to hold a cup or a mug (figure 78). China mugs are unduly heavy and may require both hands for lifting when they are filled with your drink. For me, this feels clumsy. I prefer using a drinking straw if I am served with a heavy mug, and leaving the mug on the table. I find plastic cups so much lighter and therefore easier to handle. I can easily handle plastic juice cups with one hand, and this is much more comfortable than using both hands or a straw. You can naturally also drink warm coffee or tea from such a cup. I also found plastic mugs with large handles which I can hold comfortably with one hand by slipping the middle finger, ring finger, and little finger through the handle and resting the index finger on top of handle (figure 78).
- Sometimes it is difficult for the arthritic to keep the dinner plate from moving around when cutting meat. You just may not have strength enough to press the knife down, in addition to the back and forth cutting motion. You can use a thin rubber mat under the plate to prevent it from moving. You can cut it from thin rubber sheeting available at drug stores. Another difficulty may occur when you try to fill your fork or spoon with food by pushing it on with the knife—some ar-

**78.** *We are usually advised to hold a china mug or cup with both hands. I prefer to hold a plastic mug with three fingers through the handle.*

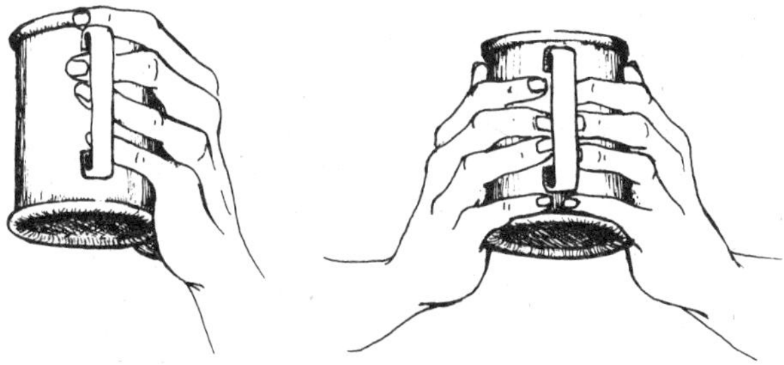

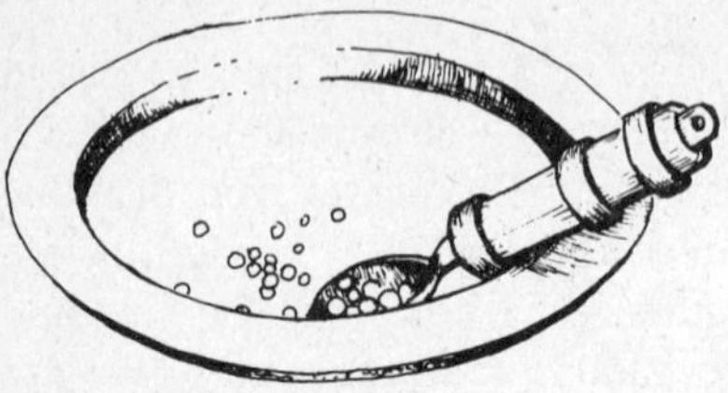

**79.** *A dinner plate with a specially deep inner lip is available as an aid to preventing food spills due to clumsiness. A foam rubber bottom prevents it from slipping. Solid white dishwasher-proof plastic 9½" (24 cm) diameter. AA 74531*

thritics do not have enough agility for this. In this case, food gets pushed to the inner lip of the plate and spills onto the rim. To solve those two difficulties, a so called inner-lip plate is available (figure 79). The extra deep inner lip is meant to prevent spills. The white plate is molded of durable polypropylene, has a 9½-inch (24 cm) diameter, is okay for the dishwasher, and the rim is one full inch (25 cm) high. A foam rubber bottom prevents the plate from slipping.

- You may build up your own spoons, forks, and knives with foam rubber or bicycle grips. If preferred, you may buy cutlery with professionally built-up handles; see Directory of Aids. The knife has a bicycle grip. The others have seven-eighths-inch (22 cm) diameter molded handles with slip rings which make handles especially comfortable to use. Figure 80 shows a teaspoon, a soup spoon, a knife, and a fork. A foam rubber adapter, one and seven-eighths-inch (4.5 cm) diameter, is available to fit over the plastic handles of the spoons and

**80.** *Cutlery is available with built-up handles. Knife is equipped with bicycle grip, others with ⅞" (22 mm) diameter molded handles. AA74620/23, SR 8AH1356/59*

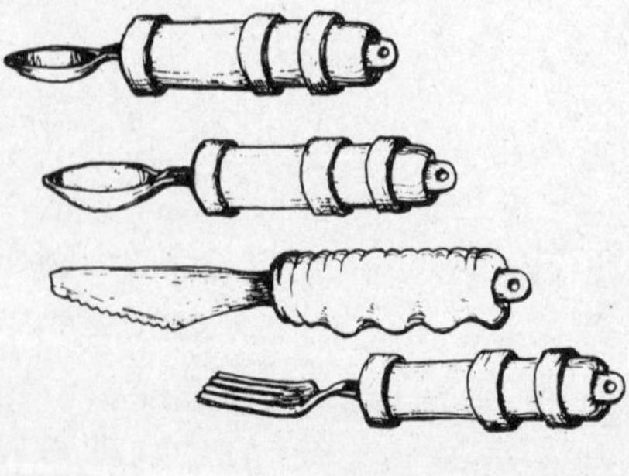

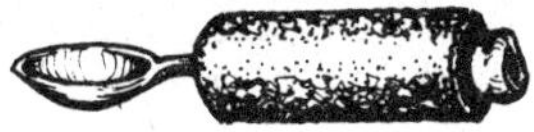

**81.** *Foam rubber adapter to fit over built-up plastic handles of spoons and forks. 1⅞" (4.5 cm) diameter, 4" (10 cm) long, available in sets of four. AA74626*

forks (figure 81). A spoon or fork with a swivel handle will make it easier for people with joint limitations to place the food into their mouth. (Available from the Independence Factory, see Directory of Aids).

## MOVING AROUND THE HOUSE

- As you move about the house, you want a comfortable chair available in every room. The most important comfort is a sufficiently high seat, so that you have no problem getting up without somebody's help and without having to lean heavily on your hands. One solution would be a tall chair in each room. These might be expensive and not fit in with your other furniture. An alternate solution is to use tall pillows. The best height is six inches (15 cm). Your upholsterer should make it with the highest density (very firm) foam rubber. A very tight-fitting covering is important. A handle permits you to carry the pillow from room to room to use on your favorite chairs. I also take my pillow out of the house. It can also be useful wherever you have to sit down—in a taxi, airplane, restaurant, doctor's office, wheelchair, etc. Isn't it wonderful to get up without having to ask for somebody's help? (Figure 82.) A professionally made device is now available: six inch (15 cm) tall pillow, very firm with zipper and handle. The pillow is 15" x 15" (38x38 cm) square.
- Adjustable bookstands are available at stationery stores. Many students use them to avoid back pain from stooping over books for long periods of time. They are useful for the arthritic at the table, especially if you sit on a tall chair, as well as in bed. Pages of a book can be turned more easily by using a rubber thimble, also available at stationery stores, for better friction against the paper.

**82.** *Now you can get up easily from a chair by using the tall pillow: 6″ (15 cm) tall, 15″ × 15″ (38 × 38 cm) square. Take it with you from room to room. Use it in a taxi, airplane, restaurant, doctor's office, etc. AA 76666*

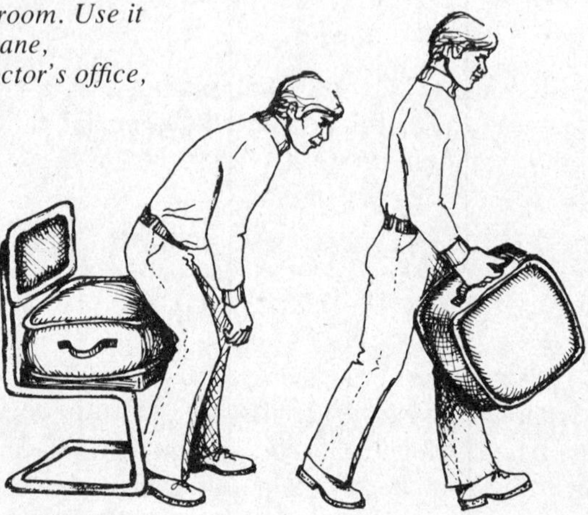

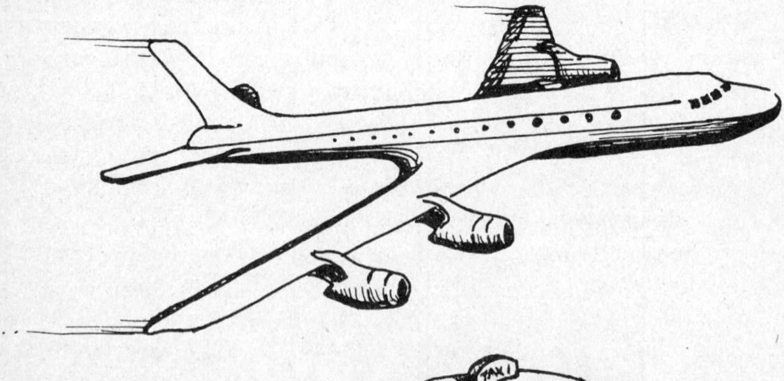

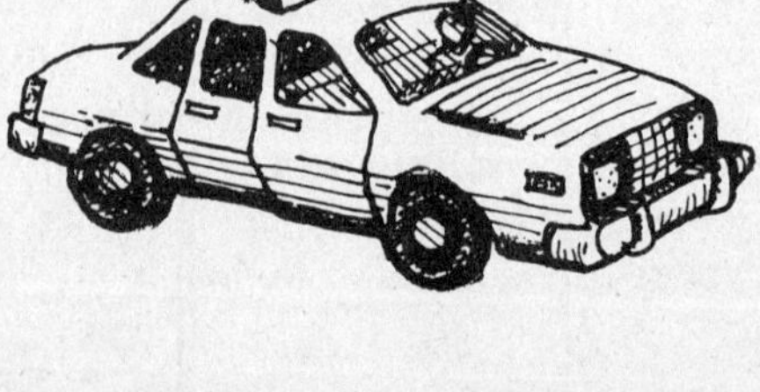

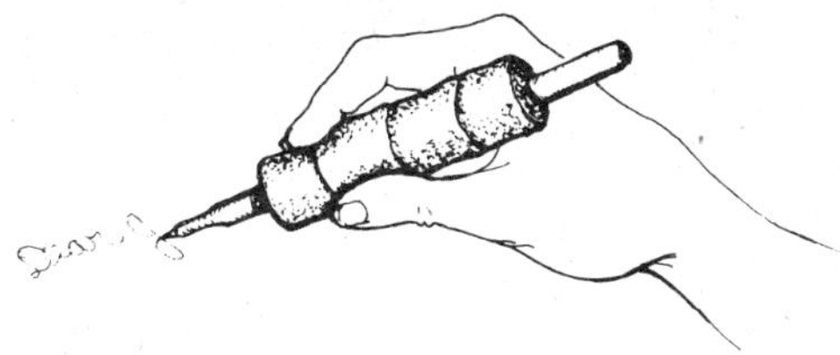

**83.** *For writing, use a smooth gliding nylon or felt tipped pen. Build up pen with foam rubber tubes from haircurlers or, for firmer grip, foam cushions from Hand Gym replacement set. AA 70902*

- Try not to lean your head on your hand. If you have to, lean on the heel of your hand so that your palm touches the face.
- Write with a pen which gives you the lightest pressure. Try a nylon or felt tipped pen. Very smooth paper gives you less friction to glide over with your pen. You may want to build up your pen with foam rubber for a more secure grip (figure 83). You can use a foam haircurler roller, or a number of foam cushions from the Hand Gym replacement set (see figure 60, page 117). Use a letter opener for your mail; do not strain your fingers.
- Typing with an electric typewriter is considered a good exercise. When typing the keys the large knuckles are kept straight. The PIP joint is flexed. IBM will sell you one of their used typewriters at cost, if you present proof of your disability. A doctor's statement is enough. There is an IBM Selectric model with a white-out correction key—very handy. There are also correcting typewriter ribbons available—upper part black, lower part white. Many typewriters are equipped for black and red ribbons. If you insert the black and white ribbon instead (available in office supply stores), you can white out individual characters, words, or sentences by depressing the red selector key and typing over the characters to be corrected. This avoids using white-out paper or ink which may be tricky for the arthritic.
- Pushbutton phones are easier to operate than dial phones. Using a ball pen held in your closed fist places less stress on knuckles when dialing. Clutching the receiver tightly during long phone conversations can result in stiff fingers, which seem not to want to let the receiver go. Get one of those

gadgets at your office supply stores which are attached to the receiver and make it easy to hold between your ear and your shoulder.

- If you watch TV you will notice that the station selector is very hard to turn. It may ruin your hands. Modern knobs are usually thin—a simple clothespin will increase leverage (figure 84).
- If you use tools, build up handles with bicycle grips for those tools requiring your strength. Foam rubber is better for precision tools with thin handles.
- If you cannot reach things which fell to the floor, use tongs to pick them up (figure 85). Using both hands strains them less. Reachers with pistol grips may be hard on the rheumatoid arthritic hands. If you have osteoarthritis the pistol grip reachers illustrated in figure 86 are very convenient to use.

## GOING OUTDOORS

- Some people find it hard to open the front door. Your hand might slip trying to turn the handle. You might wrap some plastic adhesive tape around the handle (available in the hardware store as electrical tape). Or you may prefer to buy a ready-made aid which is slipped over your handle, for increased leverage and friction (figure 87).
- I never offer my hands for a handshake for fear of having my large knuckles squashed. If somebody offers me his hand, I offer three fingers. Others usually understand right away and are gentle. In any event, they cannot compress the full arch of large knuckles (MCP joints).
- When you walk outside and use a cane, your hand may become strained leaning on the handle. Check with your surgical supply store or your therapist as to whether you should switch to a different type of handle. I am using a pistolgrip-type handle which I find easy to lean on.
- If you do not feel secure enough to walk down the tall step from the curb, try to do it walking backwards.
- If you travel, do not carry suitcases; use luggage on wheels.
- Keep small change in a European-type halfmoon-shaped

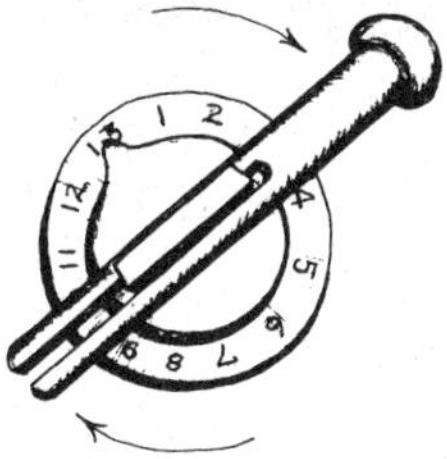

**84.** *Use a simple clothespin as an aid to turn the station selector on your TV set. May also be useful for other knobs, e.g., the small knobs of lighting fixtures.*

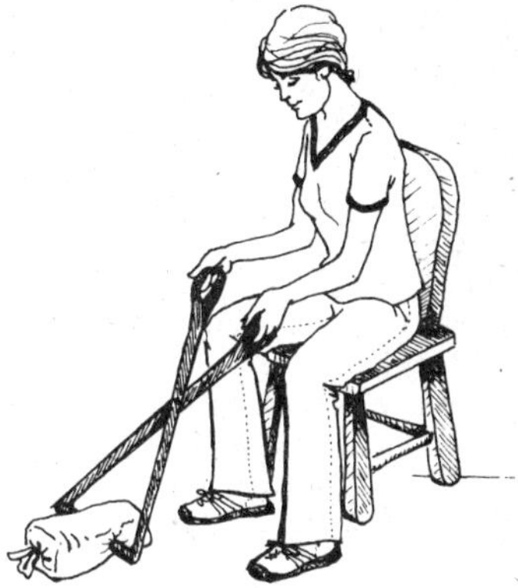

**85.** *Use tongs to pick things up from the floor. AA 72*

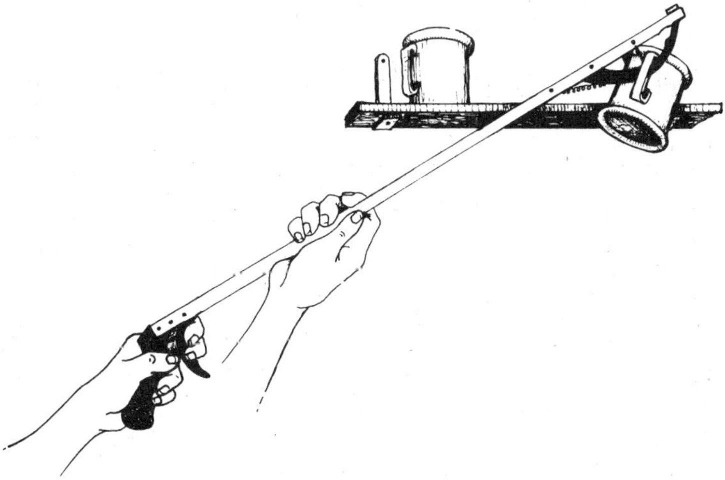

**86.** *26½" (67 cm) long pistol-grip reacher with trigger action, is lightweight and practical if you can operate the trigger. AA 76950, SR 8AH1370*

**87.** *Some adhesive electrical tape around the front door knob will give you a better grip on it. A ready-made aid gives you better leverage as well as friction. AA 7215*

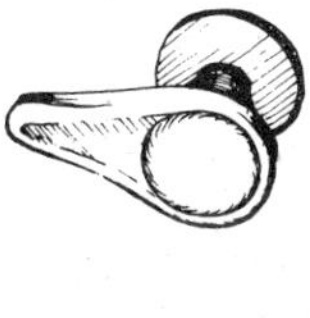

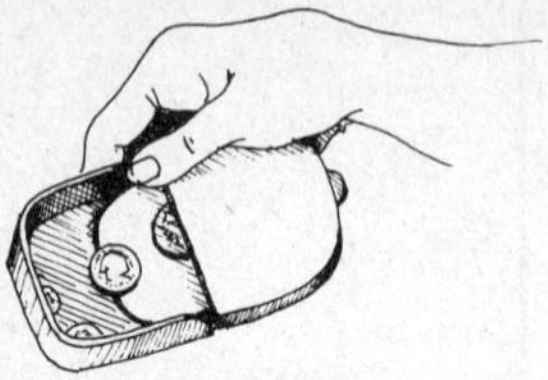

**88.** *Don't grope for coins in your pocket. Pick them up easily from the flat cover of this folding change purse.*

**89.** *A car door opener is available for opening car handles with pushbuttons; it's also good for opening recessed inside handles. AA 77382*

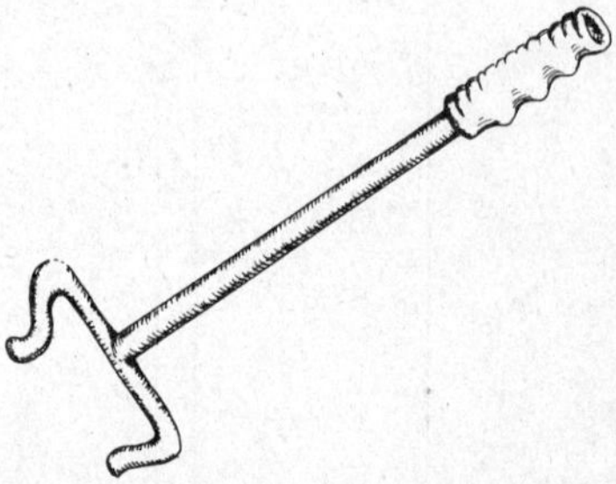

folded change purse (figure 88), available at leather goods counters. Choose a large size, to avoid having to grope for coins. They are easily picked up from the unfolded purse cover. I also find it easier to handle dollar bills when they are placed loosely in a business-letter–sized envelope in my breast pocket.

- If there is nobody there to help you open a car door, there is an aid available (figure 89). It can be used on car doors with pushbuttons and helps you obtain leverage outside and inside of any car door. See Directory of Aids.
- When you come home you may have a problem turning the key to unlock the front door. Use a very large key ring to give you extra leverage or use a commercial aid for this purpose (figure 90). See Directory of Aids.

**90.** *Use a large regular key ring for better leverage to open a door, or use a commercial holder. This one only accommodates 4 keys. AA 75412*

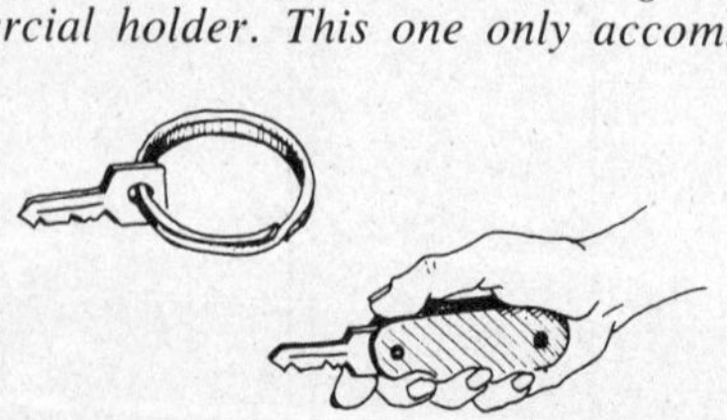

## GOING TO BED

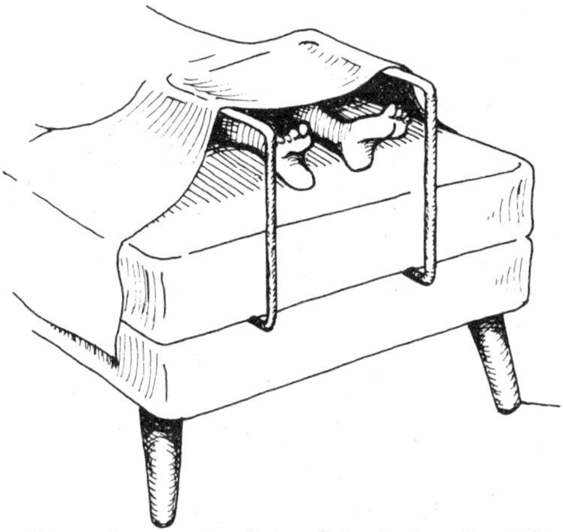

**91.** *Using this gadget at the foot of the bed makes lifting your blanket toward you easier. You feel very comfortable because it keeps the weight of the blanket off. AA 76445*

- Back at home, when you want to lie down in bed use a blanket lifter at the foot of your bed (figure 91). It will make it easier for you to pull up your blanket, with less stress on your hands. It is also beneficial to use the lightest weight blanket that provides you sufficient warmth. I found a thermal blanket or a light-weight electric blanket best for this purpose.
- Use a hand-rest splint (figure 92) to reduce inflammation and

**92.** *Hand-rest splint. Wear it at night to reduce inflammation and to control ulnar deviation if present.*

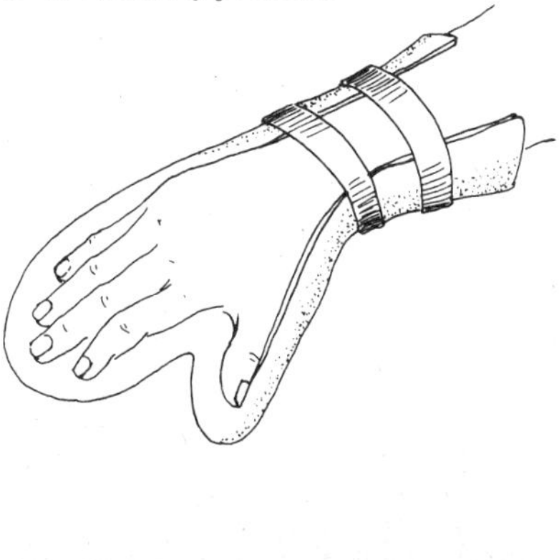

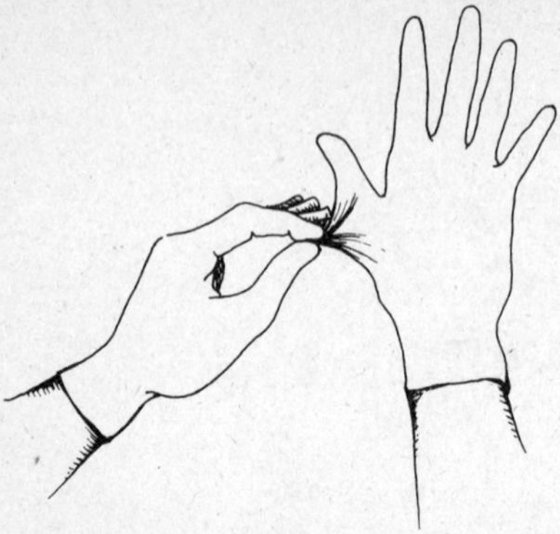

**93.** *Stretch gloves made of Lycra, nylon, and spandex may help reduce swelling of fingers and reduce morning stiffness, when worn overnight (one size fits all). AA 22766*

to control ulnar deviation. You may prefer to use stretch gloves (figure 93) overnight. They tend to reduce swelling and you may feel less stiff in the morning. These are available as Isotoner gloves in department stores (one size fits all) or you may get them from Arthritis Aid Division.

# 8
# What Hand Surgery Can Do for You

## INTRODUCTION

In the course of seventeen years of arthritis, every time I saw a rheumatologist he looked carefully at my hands, especially observed the knuckles, and asked for my complaints—such as knuckle pain, finger stiffness, weakness, problems with hand function.

If the rheumatologist has exhausted his armamentarium of medications and recommended procedures, such as exercises and other physical therapy procedures, and serious pain and discomfort still persist, he might recommend an evaluation by an orthopedic surgeon who specializes in the hand. The surgeon, who will report back to your rheumatologist, may or may not recommend an operation. Some possible recommendations the surgeon might make: (1) cortisone injections into joints; (2) synovectomy (removal of the synovium from certain joints or tendons; (3) aspiration (sucking up with a syringe) of joint fluid; (4) tendon repair; (5) tendon rerouting; (6) arthrodesis (stiffening of certain joints, or; (7) finger joint replacement with Silastic rubber implants. He may also recommend (8) splints and exercises, or just to (9) wait and see him again after a certain period of time.

I have been referred to three different surgeons in the course of my arthritis and have become quite fascinated with their expertise. One permitted me to be present to observe during several hand operations. He asked me to take photographs during operations, and I participated in some of his postgraduate teaching sessions. I have also dissected hands with my rheumatologist and read books by hand surgeons (Flatt, Zancolli) on surgery of the arthritic hand, as well as articles on the analysis of hand function (individual muscles) and arthritic deformities. Recently I attended a postgraduate symposium on "Disorders of the Hand and Wrist" at the 1981 meeting of the American Rheumatism Association together with the Arthritis Health Professions Section of the Arthritis Foundation. All this is mentioned here to assure the reader of my ability to report on the subject of what you might expect from hand surgery, although I've never had hand surgery myself, except for the surgical procedure of joint injection. I will report what I have learned from surgeons as a patient and "student," as well as what I have learned through the medical literature.

The hand is an extremely complex structure. Six to seven different tendons or muscles transverse the big knuckle (MCP) joint in order to produce the myriad of possible rapid precision finger motions we are accustomed to in daily life. A very large number of tendons, muscles, nerves, blood vessels, ligaments and bones (think, for instance, of the seven carpal bones) are constantly gliding over or next to each other as the hand moves. As a matter of fact, for proper functioning the hand relies on this constant motion for lubrication. In reality it is the constant removal of lymph through motion that insures the mobility. You will notice that every part of the body which is immobilized for a while will become somewhat stiff and has to be exercised to regain full mobility. This is especially true for the hand.

For some of the major surgical hand procedures, a very extensive exercise program before, and especially after, the operation—lasting several months—is required to obtain a real benefit from such operation. Is the patient aware and ready for this? This is one important consideration in addition to wanting relief from pain, dysfunction, and having a better-looking hand. Fortunately, not all hand procedures require such long and extensive physical therapy; ask your surgeon about the requirements in your case.

## Cortisone Injections

Cortisone injection into finger joints is usually done by a surgeon familiar with the proper directional approach of the joint space with the needle to avoid puncturing tendons, ligaments, nerves, or blood vessels—quite an art in this jungle surrounding those small joints. In my case, my rheumatologist did this very skillfully and relatively painlessly in his office. First he cleaned and disinfected the skin over the joint; then he applied a spring-loaded syringe with painkiller. This was very briefly painful, but soon the area felt numb. This was followed by the well-aimed needle reaching the joint space. I could use my hand immediately thereafter and was soon covering many papers with handwriting again without developing knuckle pain. The relief was dramatic and the knuckle unswelled—as a matter of fact, it became unusually thin. The pain and redness disappeared. The cortisone, as little as it was, helped remove symptoms from other joints of the body for a week or so.

## Aspiration of Joints

One hand surgeon told me he prefers to aspirate joints (withdraw fluid with a syringe) and at the same time inject some procaine and avoid the destructive effect of cortisone on bone and cartilage. I received a good number of finger joint injections. After a while I figured out it would be better not to provoke inflammation by overwork, and to have rest periods using the hand-rest splint for an hour between my periods of handwriting. Today, about ten to twelve years after the period when I received these joint injections, I observe myself as I write these papers by hand. I am in the so-called chronic stage of rheumatoid arthritis. My gold regimen or time, one cannot tell, leave me without inflammation. My fingers look horrible because of subluxation of the MCP joints. My hands are relatively weak, but my fingers have remained flexible due to finger-curling exercise and I have quite an endurance in writing with a fine nylon tip pen on smooth paper.

## Synovectomy

Synovectomy is the removal of the synovium, the thin skin surrounding the joint space (figure 94). It is this culprit which enlarges a millionfold during inflammation, literally pressing against the ligaments, attracting fluids, enlarging the joint and producing pain. For a while it was thought that synovectomy was the "answer" to rheumatoid arthritis. But then it was found out that the synovium grows back and the trouble can start all over again if the underlying disease process is not controlled by medication, way of life, etc. Synovectomy will not be tried unless other measures to control inflammation have failed. If synovitis persists four to six months, synovectomy will be considered. I have seen quite a few people who show the small scars on top of the MCP joints indicating synovectomies. In a crowd of sixty arthritics in an arthritis club which I addressed, I saw three people who had had this procedure and seemed very happy with the results. The operation is relatively brief unless a lot of "tightening up" has to be done around the MCP joints

**94.** *Diagram of a joint.*

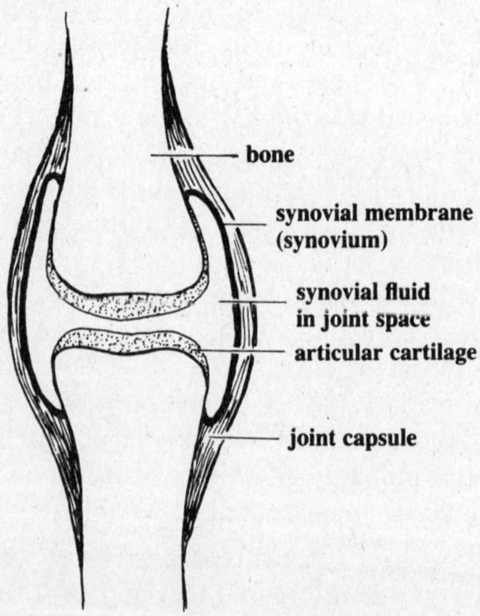

which have swollen and become loose after the operation. (My MCP joints were also swollen and then shrank after joint injections, but this procedure could not include tightening up with the result that these thin MCP joints are now subluxed due to the inability of stretched ligaments to hold the phalanges up against the power of the flexor tendons.) With the relatively short immobilization period during which I have seen patients wear functional splints with MCPs held in extension, patients seem not overly inconvenienced after the operation since they can curl their fingertips to grasp items.

Today synovectomy is done successfully around carpal bones (swelling may be visible on top of the hand). Synovium is also removed successfully from inflamed wrists with good results.

## Tendon Repair

Tendon repair refers mainly to "trigger fingers." These fingers behave in the following way: when curled, like in operating the trigger of a shotgun, the finger is stopped as if by an obstacle within the hand. When attempting to curl much harder, the finger will suddenly move, behaving much as when triggering a gun to shoot. The "obstacle" is usually swelling of the tendon which makes it stop when it hits resistance along the way.

These fingers are treated first by cortisone injections to reduce the inflammatory swellings. Such injections usually have to be repeated, as cortisone does not remove the causes but only the symptoms of inflammatory conditions. Sometimes an operation has to be performed, which consists of slitting the tendon to permit it to pass more easily through the "flexor tunnels" underneath the MCP joints. This is a minor operation, which does not incapacitate the patient for a long time.

## Rerouting of Tendons

Rerouting of tendons is a highly artistic engineering performance. If your rheumatologist refers you to a specialist for such a procedure, you can be assured that he has done many opera-

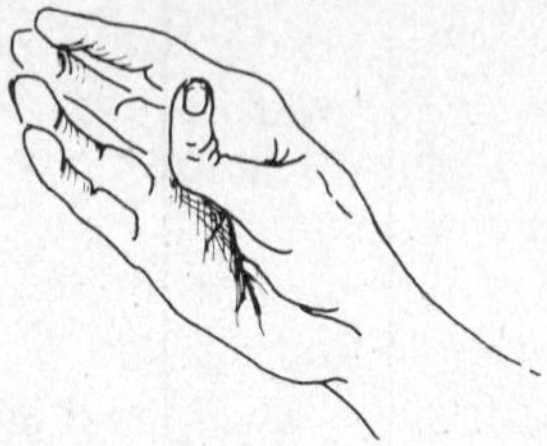

**95.** *Zigzag deformity of the thumb.*

tions and has available a qualified occupational or physical therapy team to help you obtain the best advantage from the procedure. One elegant version is to reroute the long (extrinsic) extensor tendon of the thumb (which normally only extends the distal phalanx of the thumb) to extend the proximal phalanx of the thumb, normally extended by the short extensor. Failure to extend the MCP joint of the thumb results in the typical zigzag deformity of the thumb (figure 95), which reduces pinching efficiency and eventually destroys the interphalangecal joint as it used hyperextended—rather than extended or flexed, which is the normal position for this joint. Reports by Dr. Nalebuff of Boston about his arthritic thumb reconstruction, of which I only mentioned one example, are very impressive.

When I studied anatomy I learned that there is a variety among people under the skin, not only above the skin. Some people have one vertebra more than others. I noted with interest, reading the literature on the extensor muscle of the thumb, that although most people have both the long and short extensors, a certain percentage are lacking the short extensor (extensor pollicis brevis) altogether, yet they still can extend both phalanges of the thumb to pinch normally. Surgeons like Dr. Nalebuff engineer the rerouting of tendons just as nature helps itself by compensating for missing muscles.

Another variation is to reroute a tendon from one finger to another. I will not discuss the reasoning here. The machinery of the hand is very complex. It comes into a lot of disarray during arthritis. Such rerouting, carried out surgically, may not be a major procedure. The patient will have to re-educate himself in the use of his hand, however. He will find that as he wants to lift one finger, he will instead lift a different finger. Patient work with a therapist will accomplish the necessary re-education.

## Arthrodesis

This is fusing of a joint and is usually considered after loss of cartilage. This was suggested to me for the MCP joints of both thumbs. The CM and MCP joints of my thumbs were the first joints to be involved when my arthritis broke out suddenly and violently. About three years later the typical zigzag deformity started to appear in both thumbs, making gripping and writing inefficient. The hand surgeon to whom my rheumatologist referred me suggested stiffening the MCP joints of the thumbs, so that the thumb tips would be placed into correct position for all time (figure 95a). He told me, "We do not have to do it now, but I know you will come back to me sooner or later." The surgeon's attitude was quite correct. In progressive rheumatoid arthritis conditions of this sort can only become worse and eventually require what is called reconstructive surgery. My rheumatologist referred me to another hand surgeon for a second opinion. He was not enthusiastic about stiffening the MCPs of my thumbs. He found the CM joints also slack and concluded

**95a.** *Zigzag deformity of the thumb corrected by arthrodesis: pin to straighten MCP joint.*

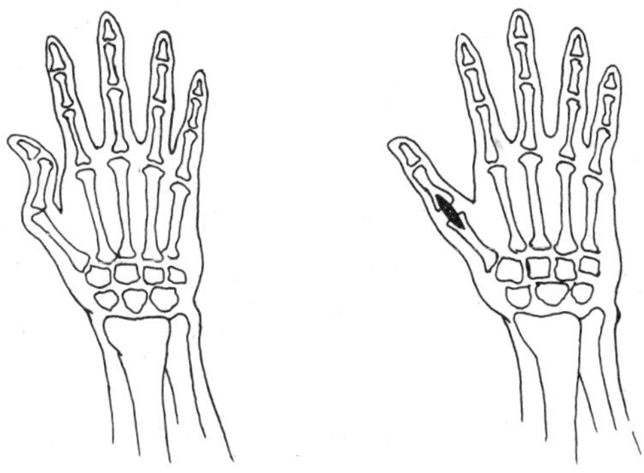

that they would deteriorate more, having to absorb the forces of stiffened MCP joints. He prescribed thumb splints which immobilized both MCP and CM joints and positioned the thumb tips properly for pinching. These splints, produced in the occupational therapy department of the hospital where the surgeon practiced, proved medically correct but inconvenient to wear. They surrounded the thumb all the way down to the CM joint and were attached tightly to the wrist. Any attempt to rotate the CM joint produced unpleasant pressure on the thumb. I found in the literature descriptions of very elegant lightweight finger splints designed by Dr. Bennett at the Warm Springs Foundation in Warm Springs, Ga. I tried to have them made in New York City and found to my amazement that no occupational therapy or orthotics department was familiar with these designs. It seems that all therapists designing splints do their own improvisations and artistry. Finally, Dr. H. R. Lehneis, director of the orthotics department of the Institute for Rehabilitation Medicine decided to copy one type of the "Bennett" splints for me in plastic. These splints extend the MCP joint and are attached to the wrist with a Velcro band, permitting rotation of the CM joint. I could discard the splint for my left thumb after a while as the joint "straightened out" sufficiently by itself (probably through adhesions) to become useful in pinching. I have been wearing the right thumb splint for many years and find it very helpful. Surgeons looking at my hands in the last year observed the splint (see figure 96) and did not suggest any surgery for the thumb.

96.

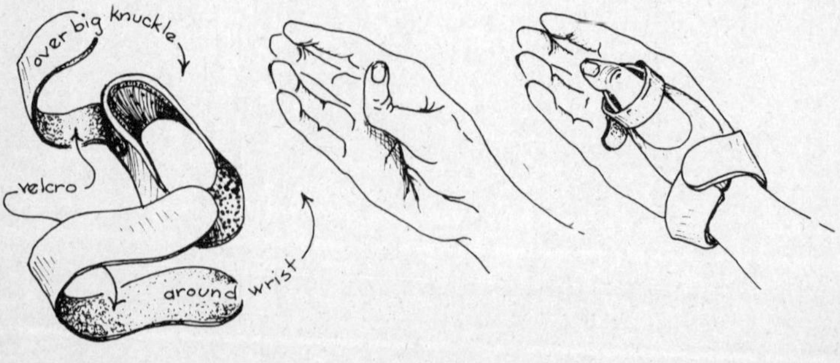

## Total Joint Replacement

Although textbooks for surgery of the arthritic hand still describe very interesting procedures, including tendon rerouting, to correct Swan-neck, Boutonniere, and Ulnar Drift deformities, the most popular reconstructive surgery today seems to be the Swanson total joint replacement (also called implant; it is named after its originator, Dr. Swanson). The implant consists of a Silastic rubber body containing two roots fitting into the metacarpal and proximal phalangeal bone respectively (figure 97). The stiffness of the rubber takes over part of the job of the extensors and intrinsics to stabilize the fingers in extension and adduction/abduction. The operation improves the flexibility of the fingers through better joint alignment and the flexibility of the Silastic rubber so that the tip of the thumb can meet the tips of the other fingers. This results in a normal-looking hand, as compared with highly distorted fingers. This is very important for the morale of the patient.

Strength cannot be expected to increase much, but this is compensated for by increased flexibility—and patients are satisfied with improved functioning and better looks.

The operation is indicated in cases of intractable pain and/or severely reduced function. I know of the wife of a physician who was a patient in a nursing home purely due to nonfunctional hands. She would undoubtedly be a candidate for this operation. I doubt that many patients will ask for this operation purely for cosmetic reasons, and few surgeons will suggest it. However, I must confess that some physicians other than my

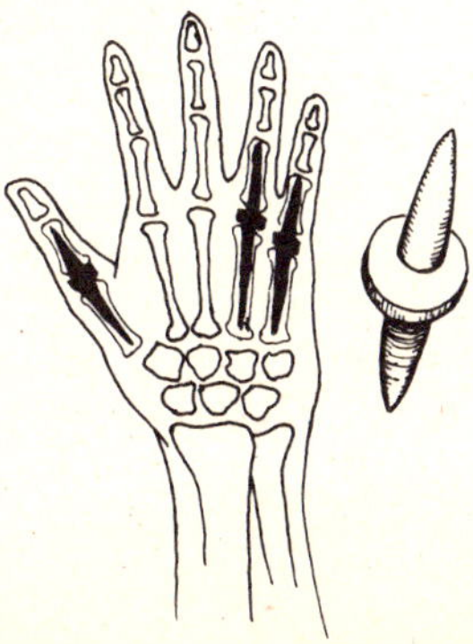

**97.** *Silastic rubber joint implant.*

rheumatologist and surgeon questioned me pointedly why I do not undergo this operation for my hands; however, although they look distorted due to subluxations, I have retained flexibility of the fingers so that I am not limited, for instance, in handling knife, fork, and writing pen. The operation would therefore not improve me functionally.

I am discussing these details to help you judge your own situation and discuss it with your physician. Ask him about the timetable of this operation, mainly regarding the exercise programs before and after and, again, a summary of results and defects of the operation which can be expected. The length of the operation and possible strain on your individual system are entirely a matter between you and your physician. I know that with the very large number of such joint replacement operations being done, the techniques are more and more perfected and present less and less strain on the patient's system.

I have read, in all descriptions of arthritis hand operations involving straightening out fingers, that the small (intrinsic) hand muscles should be stretched through exercise prior to the operation as much as possible. This will result in the largest angle through which fingers can later be actively flexed and extended. The final ''stretching'' of the fingers at the operation can only be achieved by resection (cutting) of parts of muscles or tendon fibers. Usually one or two weeks of training prior to the operation are allotted for this. I do not consider this enough time.

The Hand Gym program produced a considerable steady increase in range of motion through two to four months of exercises in the patients studied. Keep this in mind if you consider a finger joint replacement operation and do the Hand Gym program for several months prior to the operation. Make sure, however, that you can flatten your hand sufficiently so that you can assume the protective position in the Hand Gym. An occupational therapist may help you achieve this.

During the operation the head of the metacarpal bone and the base of the proximal phalanx will be adjusted to fit the implant between the two bones. See figure 97, page 147. Similarly, a smaller implant may be used for the PIP joint. After the operation the hand is immobilized for three to four weeks in an ''out-

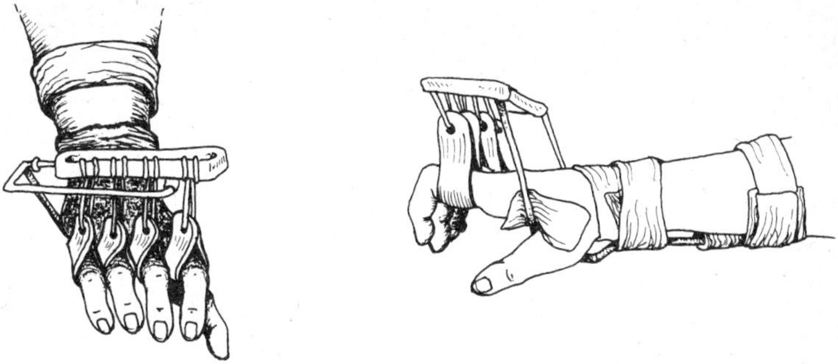

**98.** *Outrigger splint used after joint implant surgery.*

rigger splint" with the fingers suspended in the extended position for passive and, later, gentle active flexion exercises (figure 98). These are first carried out with the help of an occupational therapist. After the splint is removed, strengthening and flexibility exercises are continued for many months.

The result is a good-looking pain-free hand, more flexibility, probably no gained strength. Occasionally an implant will break, but this will be mostly tolerated and will not require further replacement. In spite of the lack of additional strength, patients seem to be satisfied with the improved functioning of their "new" good-looking hands.

Physicians from the Mayo Clinic have critically reviewed results obtained with Swanson implants and call for improvement of these joint replacements to decrease breakage and permit more improvement in strength.

It has been stated that the gains are only temporary, and after five years the disease process may again cause function to deteriorate. However, as a patient with long-standing disease myself, and as the interviews with patients on the Hand Gym in a four-year follow-up show, arthritics are grateful for all increased mobility at a point where they are losing function. They can adjust more easily to slowly decreasing strength.

# Directory of Aids

## WHERE TO BUY IT

There are virtually hundreds of mechanical aids available to help the arthritic improve his function. Many of them are imported, many of them are made in U.S.A., and many of them you can make yourself.

I wish they were as easy to obtain from your drugstore as medications—unfortunately, this is not the case. Nobody seems to stock the large variety of aids available. It may be easier for you to shop at a local department store for some items—for instance, a lightweight plastic mug with a large handle or some tongs to pick up things from the floor.

For instructions on how to make aids yourself consult: "Aids and Adaptations," $2.50 from the Canadian Arthritis and Rheumatism Society, 45 Charles St. East, Toronto M4Y153, Canada.

Your next bet to obtain self-help aids is in your medical or surgical supply store. They usually stock only a few popular items. If the salesperson is patient enough, he will let you look at one of the manufacturers' catalogs so you can select an item. Delivery may take a long time if it is not in stock at the manufacturer. You may also not be sure how the item will work out for you.

If you want to write to one of the largest manufacturers for their free catalog, the address is: Maddak Inc., Pequannock, N.J. 07440. They may also advise you of a store near you through which you can order their products.

There are two excellent manuals with hundreds of items and sources:

1. *Self Help Manual for Arthritis Patients,* published by the Arthritis Foundation, $3.00 from your local Arthritis Foundation chapter or by mail from Arthritis Foundation National Headquarters, 3400 Peachtree Road North East, Atlanta, Georgia 30326.

2. *Mealtime Manual for People with Disabilities and the Aging,* $3.50 from Campbell Soup Company, Box MM 56, Camden, New Jersey 08101.

I found these two manuals too overwhelming for my first contact with arthritic aids, but I believe they are very worthwhile for reference and ideas.

To simplify your job of obtaining devices which I have tried out myself, I have devised the list that follows, with the Sears Roebuck catalog numbers and the Arthritis Aids Division catalog numbers for each device shown in chapter 7, as well as their present prices and ordering information.

Arthritis Aids Division (AA) *absorbs* your local sales tax, shipping and insurance. For handling charges, see page 153. For prices starting January 1983, write for current catalog to Arthritis Aids Division, P.O. Box 111, Point Lookout, N.Y. 11569.

To Sears Roebuck (SR) prices *add* your local sales tax, plus parcel post charges (see page 153). For prices after February 1, 1983 obtain new Home Health Care Catalog from Sears Roebuck, Philadelphia, Pa. 19132.

The Independence Factory, 1385 Central Ave., Middletown, Ohio, 45042 publishes 3 Do-It-Yourself "Make It Cheap" manuals, 3 vol. $8.50 (machine shop needed). Catalog of reasonably priced aids available, price $1.00 (refunded with first order).

# PRICE LISTS OF AIDS

| Fig. # | Description | AA Cat. # | AA Price | Sears Cat. # | S.R. Price | S.R. Shipping Weight |
|---|---|---|---|---|---|---|
| 56 | Toilet Seat, 4″ | 72580 | 18.00 | 8AH1186 | 16.99 | 3 lbs. |
| 56 | Toilet Seat, 6″ | 72586 | 25.00 | — | — | |
| 58 | Tap Turner | 75315 | 9.00 | — | — | |
| 60 | Hand Gym Repl. Parts | 70902 | 1.50 | — | — | |
| 62 | Dental Floss Aid | 74155 | 2.85 | — | — | |
| 63 | Nail Brush | 74148 | 6.00 | — | — | |
| 64 | Wash Mitt | 74132 | 5.00 | — | — | |
| 65 | Sm. Whirlpool Bath | — | — | 8AH2262 | 34.99 | 7 lbs. |
| 66 | Hand Gym | 70900 | 20.00 | — | — | |
| 67 | Dressing Stick | 73881 | 10.00 | — | — | |
| 68 | Button Loop (sm) | 73884 | 6.00 | — | — | |
| 70 | Hose Helper | 73845 | 21.00 | — | — | |
| | Plastic Shoehorn, 17½″ (44cm) | 73824 | 2.00 | 8AH1372 | 1.99 | 2 ozs. |
| | Shoe laces (Bl.) 3pr | 73814 | 3.95 | — | — | |
| | Shoe laces (Br.) 3pr | 73815 | 3.95 | — | — | |
| 71 | No-Bows (Br.) | 73810 | 2.50 | — | — | |
| 71 | No-Bows (Bl.) | 73811 | 2.50 | — | — | |
| 73 | Un-Skru | 75346 | 5.75 | 8AH1366 | 5.99 | 2 ozs. |
| 74 | Swedish Serrated Carving Knife | 75326 | 18.00 | — | — | |
| 75 | Potato Peeler | 75330 | 5.35 | — | — | |
| 76 | Stove Valve Turner | 75433 | 12.90 | — | — | |
| 77 | Nail Brush | 74148 | 6.00 | — | — | |
| 79 | Inner Lip Plate | 74531 | 3.25 | — | — | |
| 80 | Teaspoon | 74620 | 3.50 | 8AH1356 | 3.69 | 4 ozs. |
| 80 | Soup Spoon | 74621 | 3.60 | 8AH1357 | 3.69 | 4 ozs. |
| 80 | Knife | 74622 | 5.25 | 8AH1358 | 5.99 | 4 ozs. |
| 80 | Fork | 74623 | 3.60 | 8AH1359 | 3.69 | 4 ozs. |
| 81 | Foam Rubber Adapter (Set of four) | 74626 | 2.65 | — | — | |
| 82 | Tall Pillow | 76666 | 34.50 | — | — | |
| 85 | Tongs, Wooden, 27″ | 72 | 10.98 | — | — | |
| 86 | 26½″ Pistol Grip Reacher | 76950 | 15.00 | 8AH1370 | 15.99 | 6 ozs. |
| 87 | Slip-on for Door Handle | 7215 | 5.00 | — | — | |
| 90 | Key Holder | 75412 | 4.80 | — | — | |
| 89 | Car Door Opener | 77382 | 22.50 | — | — | |
| 91 | Blanket Lifter | 76445 | 8.50 | — | — | |
| 93 | Isotoner Stretch Gloves | 22766 | 12.00 | — | — | |

**To order from AA Div.**

To total of prices of items chosen, add handling charges:

$2 if total is less than $10.00
$3 if total is less than $25.00
$4 if total is more than $25.00

Send check or money order to Arthritis Aids Div., P.O. Box 111, Point Lookout, N.Y. 11569

**To order from Sears**

1. Add prices of items wanted

2. Local sales tax

3. Parcel post charges for total weight for the distance between your location and Philadelphia, Pa. (consult your post office). Send check or money order for total to Sears Roebuck, Philadelphia, Pa. 19132

The above mail order houses stock all their items for prompt shipment.

If the amount sent is incorrect, the items will usually be shipped to you with a request for the difference due or a refund.

# Bibliography


Bennett, R. L. *Wrist and Hand Slip on Splints,* In Licht S.: Arthritis and Physical Medicine, New Haven, Elizabeth, Licht, 1969

Bens, Doris E., and Krewer, Semyon E. "The Hand Gym: An Exercise Apparatus for the Patient with Rheumatoid Arthritis." *Archives of Physical Medicine and Rehabilitation,* Vol. #55 (October 1974): 477–80.

Bland, J. H. *Arthritis: Medical Treatment and Home Care.* New York: Collier Books, 1962.

Brattstrom, Merete. *Principles of Joint Protection in Chronic Rheumatic Disease.* Chicago: Yearbook Medical Publishers, Inc., 1975.

Cailliet, Rene. *Hand Pain and Impairment.* Philadelphia: F. A. Davis Company, 1971.

Casley-Smith, J. R. *"How the Lymphatic System Works." Lymphology,* Vol. 1 (1968):77–80.

Ehrlich, George E. *Total Management of the Arthritic Patient.* Philadelphia: Lea and Febiger, 1973.

————*Rehabilitation Management of Rheumatic Conditions,* Williams & Wilkins, Baltimore, 1980.

Enrlich, G. E., and DiPiero A. M. *Stretch Gloves: Nocturnal Use to Ameliorate Morning Stiffness in Arthritic Hands.* Arch. Phys. Med. Rehab (1971):479–80.

Flatt, A. *The Care of the Rheumatoid Hand.* St. Louis: C. V. Mosby, 1974.

Fries, James, F., M.D. *Arthritis, A Comprehensive Guide.* Reading, Mass.: Addison-Wesley, 1979.

Hettinger, Theodor. *Isometrisches Muskeltraining.* Stuttgart: Georg Thieme Verlag, 4th ed. 1972.

Hollander, Joseph L., Ed. *Arthritis and Allied Conditions, A Textbook of Rheumatology.* Philadelphia: Lea & Febiger, 9th Ed. 1979.

Klinger, Judith L. for Allied Health Professions Section of the Arthritis Foundation. *Self-Help Manual for Arthritis Patients.* The Arthritis Foundation, 1980.

Krewer, Semyon E. "Calibrated Grasping Tubes for Intrinsic-Plus Testing of Arthritic Hands." *Archives of Physical Medicine and Rehabilitation,* Vol. 59 (June 1978):293–94.

Krewer, S., and Edgar, A. *The Arthritis Exercise Book*. New York: Cornerstone Library, 1981.

Lamont-Havers, Ronald W., and Hislop, Helen J., Eds. *Arthritis and Related Disorders*. New York: American Physical Therapy Association, 1965.

Lieberman, Nathan. "Your Best Dental Instrument, Your Hands; Exercises to Reduce Muscle Fatigue." *Dental Survey* (April 1973) 56–58.

MacBain, K. P.; Galbraith, M.; and Brady, F. "Non-Operative Hand Management of Adult-Onset Rheumatoid Arthritis," Vancouver, B.C.: *The Arthritis Society,* 1981.

Müller, Erich A. "Influence of Training and of Inactivity on Muscle Strength." *Archives of Physical Medicine and Rehabilitation,* Vol. 51, August 1970:449–62.

Omer, G., and Carter-Wilson M. "Disorders of the Hand and Wrists." Postgraduate Clinical Seminar, American Rheumatism Association, Boston (June 3, 1981).

Resnick, Donald, M.D. "Arthrography in the Evaluation of Arthritic Disorders of the Wrist." *Radiology,* Vol. 113, #2 (November 1974) 331–40.

Rusznyak, I.; Foldi M.; and Szabo, G. *Lymphatics and Lymph Circulation*. London: Pergamon Press, 1960.

Schaufler, Judith; Sverdlik, Samuel S.; Baker, Anita; and Krewer, Semyon E. " 'Hand Gym' for Patients with Arthritic Hand Disabilities: Preliminary Report." *Archives of Physical Medical and Rehabilitation,* Vol. 59 (May 1978) 221–26.

Sverdlik, S. S.; Simmons, A.; Krewer, S. E. "Follow-up Study of Hand Gym Exercise Program for Patients with Rheumatoid and Osteoärthritis Hand Disabilities." Presented at Annual Meeting of Academy of Physical Medicine and Rehabilitation, New Orleans (1978).

Wynn-Parry, C. B. *Rehabilitation of the Hand*. London: Buttersworth, 1973.

Zancolli, Eduardo. *Structural and Dynamic Bases of Hand Surgery*. Philadelphia and Toronto: J. B. Lippincott Co., 1968.

# Index